Coping With A Myositis Disease

Written by Myositis Patients telling their personal story of dealing with this muscle disease

Dermatomyositis - DM
Polymyositis - PM
Inclusion Body Myositis - IBM
Juvenile Dermatomyositis - JDM

With a Foreword by
- Dr. Aziz Shaibani
Nerve & Muscle Center of Texas,
Houston Medical Center

Real Life Stories
as told by Individuals with Myositis

Published by James R. Kilpatrick (IBM)
Kilpatrick Publishing Company

Kilpatrick Publishing Co.
***

Library of Congress Card Number: 00-191174
International Standard Book Number 0-97016-71-05
***

DISCLAIMER: The true life stories written with hands-on experience in this book by individuals with one of the Myositis diseases tell how they had to learn for themselves how to deal in their respective way with a life-changing disease. The information, data, facts and theories furnished herein do not reflect in any manner the medications, therapy or treatment should be considered medical advise; nor should the book be used for diagnostic purposes or diagnosis. The information in the book makes no representation, warranties, expressed or implied, by the Publisher or writers.

The stories contained herein were written exactly as the individuals expressed themselves. The stories are as they were submitted for the book.
The purpose of this book is not to be a literary work by renown people, but written just as the individuals with a Myositis disease tell other Myositis patients how they are handling the disease.
Through their experiences we hope to help other Myositis individuals and their families gain better understanding of the changes that will be made in their future.

Printed in New York City, New York, USA
***

E-Mail - JRKilpatrickMYO@aol.com

Dedication

Who else would be more qualified or deserving to have the "*Coping with a Myositis Disease*" dedication page recognition than those who wrote personally, or their caregiver, telling their own experience of handling the disease, how they and their family have learned their own methods and solutions of coping and necessary changes in their life styles when an unknown word - *Myositis* - enters uninvited into a household?

For that reason, the dedication of "*Coping with a Myositis Disease*" goes to two categories of individuals. Like the song says, "*You Can't Have One Without the Other,*" we are dedicating this book to those

(1) Having a Myositis disease and to the
(2) Care givers who are so vital to the Myositis individual

The two have to go hand in hand even when times are truly rough, when the future is bleak, when the sun looks like it will never again shine, through uncertainty and during the gains and the low points.

Speaking personally, without my wife's faithful support and caring, taking on roles and tasks she had never faced nor ever expected to face, this book probably wouldn't have been possible.

The care givers are the unsung heroes of the real life stories contained in this book. Without complaining, virtually giving up their own life, ambitions and aspirations, they have maintained a mighty force of support, strong faith, and strength when they had exhausted all they had, and their non-condemning attitude.

No one would ever ask for this disease.

May the contents of this book be an encouragement to individuals, readers and families, knowing that none of us is truly alone battling the ravages of a Myositis disease.

Thank you, our Myositis family, for your participation in making this book a reality; written by Myositis patients for Myositis patients come to fruition. At this time of publication, no book has ever been written solely by those with Myositis and how they have dealt with the disease.

To quote Dr. Aziz Shaibani, Director of Nerve and Muscle Center of Texas, Houston, medical training facilities:

"I read the Myositis stories submitted for the book. They are fantastic as I learned a lot from them. These finer details from the patient's perspective can not be found even in the most specialized textbooks. I know my patients will like it."

I would be remiss if no mention was made about a strong faith in dealing with a Myositis disease. At least 85% of the submitted stories mentioned their faith and belief in God.

James R. Kilpatrick (IBM)
Editor and Publisher

Contents

FOREWORD

Medical textbooks talk about medical disorders and medical cases, and not about the complex interaction between the medical disorders and the specific individual's psychology to produce what we call "patients."

"*Coping with a Myositis Disease*" does not only talk about patients but also written and edited by patients, thus providing a unique contribution to the medical and public library alike.

James R. Kilpatrick (IBM) has made admirable personal efforts to make this book available and affordable to many patients whose budgets are already exhausted by their limited physical fitness and the financial demand of treating and coping with Myositis.

Psychological and physical adaptation to acute and subacute disorders such as Polymyositis and Dermatomyositis are not the same when the disorders are chronic such as Inclusion Body Myositis (IBM), and in both cases, people vary in their techniques and strategies to cope with these disorders. This book, therefore, provides patients with a variety of ways and resources; thereby patients could "trick" the disease and minimize its impact on their life; something doctors cannot do.

Inflammation muscle diseases is not a uniform group of muscle disorders. Polymyositis is an autoimmune muscle inflammation that is more common in women. Dermatomyositis is an inflammatory disorder of the intramuscular blood vessels and affect women more than men of different age groups. While Inclusion Body Myositis is a chronic disorder of mostly older men and it is the most common muscle disease or a degenerative disorder like Alzheimer disease (some experts call it Alzheimer's disease of the muscle); very interestingly many molecules removed from muscles affected with IBM are identical to those recovered from brains of patients with Alzheimer's disease.

Polymyositis and Dermatomyositis usually respond to treatment very well (steroids, cytotoxic drugs, intravenous gammaglobulin, etc), while IBM does not, unless diagnosed eary. The average duration between the onset of symptoms and the diagnosis of IBM is 8 years, partly because of lack of public awareness of the symptoms and the disease and partly because of the delayed referral to the neuromuscular specialists by the primary care doctors either because of lack of awareness again or because of the strict HMO gate-keeping rules or both.

Retrospectively, many of my IBM patients report they had to change their lifestyle years before they sought medical advice, many stopped dancing because their knees would unbuckle, leading to falls in public. Others thought they were just out of shape.

I hope "*Coping with a Myositis Disease*" will be used for fund raising or other activities to increase the public awareness of the symptoms of Myositis.

Finally, I think patients will appreciate finding this book in the reception areas of neuromuscular and rheumatological clinics.

—*Dr. Aziz Shaibani, Director*
Nerve & Muscle Center of Texas
Houston, Texas

Myositis

Myositis refers to inflammation of the muscles (*Myo* means muscle and *itis* means inflammation) Myositis is a term that describes several different diseases, including

Dermatomyositis - DM
Polymyositis - PM
Inclusion Body Myositis - IBM
Juvenile Dermatomyositis - JDM

Polymyositis means *inflammation of many muscles.*
Dermatomyositis means *inflammation of muscle and skin*
Inclusion Body Myositis means *inflammation of the muscles with Inclusion (abnormal protein deposits) and vacuoles (holes) in the muscle cells and fibers.*

All forms of Myositis usually involve chronic, or persistent, muscle inflammation; almost always result in weakness of muscles, falling down frequently, sometimes swelling feet and legs, loss of strength and pain of the muscles and joints for many with the disease.

Early indications of inflammation of the muscles may

* Include difficulty in rising from a chair, climbingsteps, or lifting the arms and began experiencing falling at random.
* Become exceedingly fatigued after prolonged standing or walking.
* Loss of strength throughout the body is experienced.
* For some, difficulty in swallowing and breathing becomeslabored; also, the voice may become raspy and hoarse sounding.

It is estimated each year 5 to 7 out of every million people get a form of Myositis annually.

Although Myositis can affect people of any age, most children who get the disease are between five and 15 years of age and most adults are between 30 and 60 and over. Like many other inflammatory diseases, most forms of Myositis attack more women than men. The exception is Inclusion Body Myositis (IBM), a form of Myositis in which inclusions (abnormal protein deposits) and vacuoles (holes) develop in the muscle fibers. This form of Myositis affects more men that women.

No one is sure what causes Myositis. But because Myositis has many forms, it probably has many causes. Some scientists think that Myositis may result when a person with a certain genetic background is exposed to particular chemicals, viruses, or other infectious agents. All medical professionals do not agree with this accessment.

A physician will run a battery of tests while processing a diagnosis; asking the patient many questions; complete physical exam, blood tests for numerous diseases or factors; including a blood test for muscle enzyme called *creatine kinasis* or CK, maybe a spinal tap, and electromyogram (EMG), a MRI and a muscle biopsy. It may be necessary to repeat many of the tests and biopsies.

The treatments and medications vary from person to person and will change as the disease progresses. A therapy or mediation recommended by one physician may vary from that of another physician. Considerations of the severity and type of problems have to be taken into account as each person's situation is not the same with another, even both may be diagnosed as having the same Myositis disease.

CORTICOSTEROIDS: Virtually, every physician's first prescription is Prednisone. The drug helps with DM, PM, JDM, and to some limited extent, IBM at first, but often times creates more problems in other areas of the body than expected: weight gain, moon face, moon barrel chest, moon belly, depression, cataracts and diabetes.

Anyone taking corticosteroids should be monitored carefully by their physician and should report any new medical problems to the physician.

Some physicians will include other immunosuppressants or corticosteroids which may or may not help every patient.

IMMUNOSUPPRESSANTS: If a patient does not respond to Prednisone favorably, other drugs called immunosuppressants (the commonly used for Myositis are Methotrexate and Azathioprine) are used. These drugs slow down the immune system, reducing its ability to attack infections and attack healthy tissues in persons with autoimmune diseases.

Immunosuppressant drugs are powerful and can result in side effects such as upset stomach, loss of appetite, mouth sores, hair loss, skin rash, chills and fever, diarrhea and other problems for some patients.

Myositis, like most other forms of muscle disorders is a chronic disease. It affects every person differently. Some people have remissions and flares which may or may not last for a long time. At resent, IBM patients have little-to-no option of specific medications.

Internet Links of Interest

These web sites offer information for further information of the Myositis diseases and/or related conditions:

www.hospitaldirectory.com Hospital and Physicians
www.ama.assn.org/aps/amahg.htm Provides information on virtually every licensed physician in the U.S.
www.familydoctor.org A searchable library from the American Academy of Family Physicians
www.nih.gov National Institute of Health
www.medicinenet.com Site includes medical dictionary, references, links and news
www.medscape.com One of Internet's biggest collection of peer-reviewed articles
www.ninds.nih.gov Site on Nat'l Library of Medicine
www.neurologychannel.com Neurology & Neuromuscular
www.americanscooters.com Scooters at wholesale price
www.pridehealth.com Pride scooters and chairs
www.access-able.com Getting out and about
www.aarda.org American Autoimmune site
www.usdoj.gov/crt/ada/adahome1.htm Americans with Disabilities Law
www.ssa.gov Social Security Administration
www.nhpco.org Nat'l Hospice & Palliative Care
www.arthritis.org Arthritis Assoc.
www.mdausa.org Muscular Dystrophy Assoc.
www.myositis.org Myositis Association of America
www.rheumatic.org Rheumatic Group
www.accordent.com

This bears repeating: Research holds the key to better ways to prevent, diagnose, and control Myositis.

The Importance of Care Givers

The most important person in the life of a Myositis patient is the caregiver. It's not the physician the patient sees for a few minutes every few weeks, but it is the constant 24-hour day care the caregivers must provide.

If the man becomes the patient, he is nurtured and supported by his caregiver, most likely his wife. Both are thrown into a situation that neither asked for and neither expected to happen.

A woman soon realizes that the responsibility of maintaining the house, cleaning, cooking, laundry, caring for her husband as he gets more dependent when she has to lift him out of bed, into a chair, bathe him, dress him, drive him to the doctor, and take care of his personal hygiene can very quickly become overwhelming.

The vacuum hasn't been run in weeks, the laundry is piled up, dishes stacked in the sink - all because she doesn't have the time for anything except for the care of her husband.

Maybe she has never had any financial responsibilities but now finds herself practically alone with a check book with a small balance, a handful of bills, a leaking water pipe, a leaking roof, a strange noise in the car's engine and weeds overtaking the lawn.

If the man is the caregiver, his lack of knowledge of household duties quickly becomes apparent. The soiled linens, towels, clothing are insurmountable and he has no idea how to get the washing machine running. The kitchen had always been off bounds to him, but he learns that it is his responsibility to cook for himself and his wife. No one, sick or well, can survive forever on hot dogs, colas, chips, hamburgers, and frozen dinners. Thankfully, the directions are on the package how to cook in the microwave.

He learns real quickly that he has the responsibility of bathing his wife, providing fresh clothes, a clean bed, combing her hair, applying a dab of makeup. He learns what is involved in getting a bra and slip on his wife for her visit to the physician.

The bills have to be paid, he can't leave his wife in her condition and he can't afford to hire an adult day sitter. The flower beds have been over taken by weeds, the sun has killed the lawn so that is one less worry to handle.

THE PHYSICIAN REPORTS that an electric scooter or wheel chair is necessary now as a safety precaution and for mobility. How can we afford something like that; how can we move it from the house to the physician's; the doors in the house are too narrow and the steps look scary? The car won't hold such bulky items. The mountain of problems seem to escalate higher and higher.

It is time to make some drastic decisions:

* Remodel the house to enlarge the doors, to make the bathroom accessible, build ramps so there will be no steps to climb or having to lift the wheel chair or scooter.

* Buy a smaller house that requires little maintenance work, but it means getting rid of Grandma's furniture. What to do with all the clothes? New houses don't have the space like the larger, older homes.

* Or maybe a better solution would be to move into a Senior adult community where each home is built to comply with the ADA laws, where no maintenance or yard work is required. Such communities usually have park-like areas with paths through the trees and grounds.

Time to trade in the old Chevy and buy something reliable that a scooter or wheel chair can be hauled? But which? What? So many choices, so little time, so much to do. Where does it all end?

Although this is but a glimpse into what the future may hold, tough decisions must be made, if not now, then sometime in the future. These decisions must be made while both patient and caregiver can express their thoughts.

A current will?
Full financial knowledge of every source?
Access to the financial matters?
Directive to Physician signed?
Power of Attorney signed?
General Power of Attorney signed?

Life Insurance beneficiaries as wanted?

Learn to talk about the possibility of death and any special requests that are wanted, what plans to be made?

Caregiving is more than becoming a mechanical robot in duties and responsibilities, void of personal feelings. Caregiving includes the humanities - listening, not just hearing; hear with the heart of what is not being said as must as what is being said. The caregiver learns to read eyes, reactions, moods, the color and texture of the skin, the voice and body motions.

If a patient moans sometimes in pain, caregivers need not ask what's hurting. A Myositis patient can't tell when/where pain is localized. The pain covers all the joints and muscles.

Learn that sitting in silence can be golden sometimes, rubbing skin lotion on all exposed areas can soothe the mind as well as the body.

Myositis diseases may cause times of restlessness, aggravation, agitation, moodiness, sarcasm, insecurity and vulnerability at times - but without a rebuttal each time, these negative factors will evaporate by themselves into a vapor.

Never forget the importance of the human touch; it surpasses any other form of communication.

This list could be amplified many times over and would never be complete. Speaking as a certified Hospice volunteer counselor for 13 years to AIDS patients, it became prime importance that each aspect of life (and dying) be in correct order.

There are many medical catalogs available for every item any ill person would ever need in their home, costing about half of what the storefront medical aid stores charge. The caregiver soon learns the importance of finances.

Chapter 1

DERMATOMYOSITIS

Dermatomyositis (DM) is the most easily recognized of the inflammatory Myopathies due to it's distinctive rash. This rash occurs as a patchy, dusky, reddish or lilac rash on the eyelids, cheeks, and bridge of nose, and on the back or upper chest, elbows, knees and knuckles. Some people with DM develop calcified nodules or hardened bumps under the skin.

Muscle weakness usually develops over a period of weeks but may develop over months or even days. The weakness initially affects those muscles closest to and within the trunk of the body, including the neck, hip, trunk and shoulder muscles. Difficulty swallowing occurs in at least one third of DM patients. Whereas less than 25% of adults report muscle pain, more than 50% of children with DM complain of muscle pain and tenderness.

Dermatomyositis can occur at any age from childhood to adulthood and is more common in females than males.

High dose Prednisone (an immunosuppresant) has been an effective treatment for many patients. Other immunosuppressants such as Azathioprine and Methotrexate are used. Unfortunately, these drugs have adverse side effects, especially after prolonged use. For some patients who do not respond well to Prednisone, intravenous administration of immunoglobulin (IVIg) has helped some patients, but is very expensive - $8,000-$12,000 or more per infusion.

Myositis is registered with the Muscular Dystrophy Association as a neuromuscular disease as well as a rheumatic disease with the Arthritis Foundation.

DM Case # 1

Diagnosed March 1998
Female - Present Age 49

I want to tell my Dermatomyositis story, hoping it may help others. I had symptoms about eight years and the doctors kept saying it was just my nerves.

When I became really sick with the disease, my Mother was dying of breast cancer that had spread to her bones. I had been taking care of her for almost a year and a half before the doctors finally diagnosed my illness correctly.

I was also working part time. The stress of watching my Mother slowly die was the hardest and most heart breaking horror I hope no one will ever endure. My Mother and I were best friends. I am now 49 years of age.

I could not stop to take care of myself or even think of myself when I was so sick. My husband, Rob, is an angel sent from Heaven. He took care of me and helped me to come to cope with the death of my Mother and the illness I was facing.

The first doctor I went to, after going about eight months, ran several blood tests and called me at work to say she was almost sure I had Lupus. The stress of that news was more than I could handle. I was so mad at the doctor calling me with the bad news at my job. I never returned to that doctor.

My family doctor called a specialist for me. He knew right away just by looking at my hands and chest what I had. Then dozens of more tests were run. For months and months I lived in terror, thinking the absolute worst possible ending to this illness. I had no one to talk to. The doctor would say, "Oh, don't worry about anything. You are going to be fine. We have several medications to try on you."

I asked him how many people did he know that has gone into remission. He said, "None." No one had ever been cured or into remission and I was not to worry? I was in such pain I could hardly walk. My arms ached all the time. My poor skin looked like I had burned myself with scalding water.

At work (and, by the way, I had 15 years of experience working in Travel), I received my annual review which was all positive and the manager put it into writing I was an exceptional employee.
About two months later, the manager called it "down sizing" and I was without a job. That was March 1999 and I have not worked since.

Thank God for the Internet. I found a wonderful lady - her name is Ruth - and she posted a message on the Myositis Association of America's Bulletin Board, telling her story of being ill with the same disease for 17 years. She would be happy to talk to any new person, to give them hope and encouragement she had learned. She has been a God-send. Most importantly, I found someone with the same disease and they were ALIVE and FUNCTIONING as a whole person.

In our area, we have absolutely no support groups or any kind of help for each other. There is very little interest in support groups even on the Internet. Through Ruth, I found other people and we started talking. Within a year I found others. After reading the MAA's *The OutLook* quarterly publication, I learned they needed a Representative for Indiana. I searched my heart and decided to give it my best.

Never in a million years would I have thought to be in this position. But this has been a blessing and I only hope through God's help (and I know He has led me to this responsibility) to help others who are sick with this disease so they will feel like they are not alone.

I know how hard it is to get out of bed when my legs and hips hurt and I can barely raise myself. I can only walk short distances and lift very light things. Everyone with DM I have talked to has stomach and colon problems. Each day, it is a struggle to manage through and act as if nothing is wrong. I pray daily for a medical break through, not only for myself, but for all those who have a Myositis disease.

It is very hard to see the weight gain from lack of energy and taking Prednisone. When we go to ball games, I struggle to walk up a few flights of steps and people look at me as if I would lose some weight, I would feel better. I wish it were that simple.

I know that my illness has been rough on my husband. I am no longer the active person he married and my career is gone. I struggle every day to feel better and not to be depressed.

We hope and pray we will not become a burden on our families and those we love.

DM Case # 2

Diagnosed June 1998 - Female - Present Age 50

CURRENT STATUS: I am one of the very fortunate and am currently healthy!

I began to feel poorly about 1992. I didn't know why it hurt to stay in one position for any length of time and why I could never stay in bed a whole night without my upper back aching. About this same time, I began to be so tired I'd come home from work and nap before taking on my normal role as mother and wife. I must note also that I was under a great deal of personal stress at this time.

I went through extensive testing at a nearby university hospital and my condition continued to deteriorate. I was wrongly diagnosed with Hereditary Coproporphynia and treated for that over the next few years. In the spring of 1998, following an outbreak of shingles, I began to experience excruciating pain in my arms and back. It became impossible for me to comb my hair without lowering my head - my arms just couldn't go that high. I couldn't reach back for my seat belt in the car or up to straighten a tangled bra strap!

I remember soaking in a bathtub to try to ease the pain and then realized that I couldn't get out of the tub! I was afraid! I couldn't reach my toes; had great difficulty putting on socks and even worse of all, I couldn't get out of bed without hooking a foot under the bed rail and roll to the floor, then trying to gather my feet beneath me and leverage myself up.

I remember looking up at the phone that had been so close at hand during the night, now being totally out of reach as I lay on the floor. At the time, I was living alone and I learned to do whatever I had to survive. Number One: *Don't lie on my stomach for fear of suffocating as I couldn't lift my head.*"

An astute physician recognized the symptoms immediately. Not only was I experiencing the muscle problems, but my hands and neck, which had remained red for several years, gave him the additional clues he needed. He ordered a CK which came back as 3213. He then ordered a muscle biopsy and started me on Prednisone. He told me it was a very serious disease and that mortality rate was five years! I was terrified!

When the biopsy confirmed his diagnosis, I took myself back to the university hospital and a specialist more familiar with the disease. I am proactive and refused to accept a five year death sentence!

Since that time, Azathioprine was added to the Prednisone and slowly I was taking less Prednisone. I have maintained a daily dose of two multiple vitamins, 1200 mg Calcium, desiccated liver tabs, 400 mg Vitamin E and CoQ10 (the latter three was my own remedy!) My hair began to fall out as these medicines and vitamins combined. At one point, I asked the question, "Was it a choice of mobility or hair? I chose mobility.

In addition to the medicines, I had weekly and sometimes bi-weekly Shiatsu massage. During these sessions, the therapist kneaded the muscles to bring in fresh blood and stretched as much as I could endure for mobility. It wasn't the usual type massage a "normal" person would experience. It was an hour of significant pain that I needed in order to get better!

My doctor doesn't like to use the term "remission" with this disease and me, but I use it freely. I have learned my limits and not to over exert either my muscles or my endurance. Yet, I try to keep my own yard, climb out of bed and get to work (sometimes it means up and hour early to work through the pain) and I guard my health as I know I am very fortunate, compared to this disease. But I also know that could change tomorrow.

DM Case # 3

Diagnosed about 1974
Male - Present Age 28

I was diagnosed when I was 2.5 years old. One physician in my hometown thought that I needed corrective shoes. The other physicians didn't know what was wrong, but they all knew that something was definitely wrong.

My parents finally found a pediatric Neurologist who diagnosed me. The first person to notice was the lady in the nursery at the church. She told my parents that I wasn't keeping up with the other boys and girls in the class; that I was slower and I didn't like getting bumped

I hurt and didn't want to play with them because I might be touched. The teacher held a me a lot. The doctor put me on Prednisone and I stayed on that for the next ten years of my life. When I was 12, I told my parents I didn't think I needed it anymore. My dad said to quit taking it and we would see what happens. I was fine except for a few episodes of weakness like not being able to do pushups and having trouble holding my arms over my head from a lying down position and even having trouble lifting my arms up to my head.

Believe it or not, but just putting my arms up over my head wore me out. My legs are very weak even to this day. I not only have Dermatomyositis but I have calcium deposits all over and inside my left leg which I have had numerous surgeries to remove it all the way back since I was 8 years old. The calcium surfaces itself begins like a pimple and ends up leaving a sore, looking much like a leper, I would imagine.

I've been using a Band-aid on my elbow for over two years now and started using a second Band-aid about a year ago because the calcium surfaced to the skin and if I don't keep it covered, it will become infected.

I have had calcium deposits removed from my buttocks, my collarbone, my knee, ankle and I do not take any medication at this time and haven't really taken any thing for Dermatomyositis probably for the past 15 years or so.

What keeps me going? Friends and more friends. I have to keep upbeat and do my best to have a positive attitude.

My parents raised me in church and I still attend. I know that without God's help, I would probably be dead by now. He gives the strength and power to do what we have to do.

I pray, not as much as I should, and prayer certainty helps. I should be dead and unable to get up out of the bed each day, but I don't want that. I have to fight as hard as I can at times, but never give up.

I learned my limitations growing up. I have a passion for football and sports. I would ask my dad why I couldn't play football like my big brothers. Tears would come to his eyes as he would tell me that I couldn't do that.

I learned what I could

and couldn't do as I became older. I played football and basketball around the neighborhood.

Sometimes I would fall down on my school work because I would be in the hospital for two weeks having surgery to remove calcium. My friends would come see me and the church always sends cards and balloons.

Growing up, I got to snow ski, water ski, swimming, bicycling and almost whatever I wanted to go and do. I think that for the most part I am in remission except when I was very small. I have very little biceps muscle and have no rear end.

Personally, I think I must look like the pictures of the POW's; just saying that is the way I think I look to everyone.

I hope my personality covers for my looks, which is what counts anyway. I am married and have two sons and are expecting our third son in two months.

Even though I don't have the figure I desire, but there are lots of people God has been merciful to like me. I don't complain. We should be thankful in all things is what the Lord says and it doesn't help if you whine and complain anyway.

Keep your chin up and fight to do what you want to do.

(Editor's note: A healthy, beautiful daughter was born in April 2000. All's well!)

PM Case # 4

Diagnosed 1987 - Female - Present Age 36

I am a 36-year-old female, diagnosed with Dermatomyositis in July 1987, at the age of 23, just a few weeks before my 24th birthday.

In January of 1987 I discovered I had Raynauds Phenomenon, which was the beginnings of my problems.

By May, I noticed a de-crease in strength and flexibility. I did not, however, tell my family doctor about this. He had scheduled an appointment for me to see a Rheumatologist regarding the Raynauds and I thought maybe arthritis was setting in.

Little did I know it was worse!

Many days I would leave work and just start crying because I was so scared. I didn't know what was wrong with me and I didn't want to know.

Finally, the day came when I would see the Rheumatologist. When I got to his office, I could hardly walk on my own. I felt like I was 100 years old. I could only shuffle along and had to ask my sisters, who came with me, to not walk so fast.

I finally told the doctor everything that was wrong. I would fall trying to get dressed. I couldn't tie my shoes. I got stuck in the bathtub and my sister had to help me out. I had trouble swallowing and was losing weight. I also had difficulty driving my car, which was a standard shift and needed help getting up from the couch or out of a chair.

The doctor was a God-send. He diagnosed me immediately but did tests to verify it. I had tubes of blood taken, an EMG, which I wouldn't wish on my worst enemy. And a biopsy. The diagnosis of Dermatomyositis was confirmed.

He placed me on 60 mg/d Prednisone for two weeks and then tapered it. My CPK at the time of diagnosis was about 8000. There was quite a bit of muscle damage and my doctor told me that if I had waited much longer, it would have been irreparable.

I felt as if a huge weight had been lifted from my shoulders. Now I know there was actually something physically wrong with me and it wasn't my imagination. I was only out of work for a week while the incision healed from the biopsy

On top of this, I had started a new job in January and was still under the waiting period for the health insurance. The insurance company refused to pay for anything.

I just couldn't believe it. They had decided that the disease must have been a preexisting condition and would therefore not cover anything related to it. I had started physical therapy before I knew this and the bills from the hospital, doctors, and the- rapists started coming in. I was on the phone with them constantly to get this covered. I just kept getting the run around.

Finally, almost one year later, my father put his foot down and contacted the family lawyer. I brought everything with me when I met with him. The lawyer said the costs should be covered. He sent several letters to the insurance company. They finally agreed to pay for everything. That was truly a blessing.

I had to admit that I was scared about what the future would be like for me. I was only 24 and had looked forward to the day I would get married and have a family. All that changed. Now, I was scared that no man would ever want me because of the disease. If I were lucky enough to find someone, could I have children?

These thoughts plagued me quite a bit though I thought I had a strong faith in God. I knew He was in control and would get me through all this trial, but I still had my fears. Throughout the next few years things went fairly smoothly. I continued working full time. My sister and I got an apartment of our own and I was independent.

Five years later, I met a man who accepted and loved me with all my problems. He even said if I couldn't bear children, we'd try adoption!

He was the answer to my prayers. We were married in July 1992.

Two months later I snapped a tendon in my right hand

and had to have surgery. It was caused by Prednisone. I have since lost a lot of function and mobility in my hand due to the surgery and the fact that healing is a problem with this disease.

But I continued on.

In March 1993 I discovered I was pregnant! What a blessing, but, again, I was scared. My doctor wasn't sure what would happen, but he was very encouraging. During the pregnancy, I felt wonderful. I had more energy than I had in years and the disease was stable.

I was on 5 mg/d Prednisone and our son was delivered prematurely. He was born with cleft lip and palate and had other premature problems. Today, he is a healthy, active six year old.

In June of 1995, I was pregnant again. I was so excited since my first pregnancy went so well. This one did not.

I was sick about the first month on. I lost weight and could barely eat anything. I had gastritis attacks and was miserable. At 32 weeks, I entered the hospital, bleeding. I was there two weeks then back home on bed rest for the remainder of the pregnancy.

In March 1996, at 38 weeks, I delivered a healthy son who is now four years old. Both our sons are miracle children since I thought I would never have any of my own.

After the second pregnancy, my husband and I decided that would be it. No more children. My doctor told us another pregnancy would be worse and could put the baby and me at risk. Plus, I don't think I would have the energy to keep up with three kids!

In July 1996, I had a severe gall bladder attack and had to have it removed. The doctors are not sure if the attack is disease related, but I tend to think that it was.

Today, I am fairly healthy and enjoy my family. I try to stay active to keep from being so stiff all the time. Still, I have my fears as what the future holds and if the disease will be passed on to my sons. I've been told it is not likely to happen, but I still worry.

The main thing that keeps me going is my faith in God. Without Him, I know I would not be where I am today, for

"He is my Rock and my Salvation."

Whenever I feel afraid, I pray to God and I know He is with me.

DM Case # 5

Diagnosed 1996 - Female Present Age 49

I knew something was wrong with me about six or seven years prior to becoming sick, before the doctors knew exactly what the sickness was.

I had strange symptoms - like my neck would burn as if I had burned myself. If I walked outside in the sun, I would become extremely sick to my stomach. I did not have the energy other people had. I know my family looked at me as if I were lazy.

I have to fight every day not to be depressed and sometimes I lost.

In the beginning, I had terrible pain in my legs and arms. They are better today. Now I fight everyday to be able to eat something that will not cause extreme indigestion, which the doctors think is caused from the medicine I am taking to stay alive, which is Prednisone.

For a very long time my husband really believed I would beat this disease with herbs and vitamins. He has always wanted to go to Disney World. We would go every day as soon as the park opened and stay until it closed. Now, I can hardly walk for an hour, if that! I feel old and afraid most of the time. Illness has made a prisoner of me. I can not hold a job. I feel all right for a couple weeks which gives me false hopes. Then I wake up and something is causing me to be sick again.

For almost a year from beginning taking the medications, I was losing my hair. I couldn't stand looking at myself. I was once beautiful, but not anymore. My hands are scarred. I walk like an old person and I am over weight from the medication and lack of energy.

What I fear the most is my husband getting tired of loving a sick person who has become a burden.

Everyday I pray to God that He will strengthen me and touch me with His healing hand.

DM Case # 6

Diagnosed 1990
Female - Present Age 56

Ok, here's my story. I am a 56 year old female and have Dermatomyositis. I was officially diagnosed in the Spring of 1990.

I first became ill during November 1972.

My first symptoms were having problems walking up and down a flight of stairs, getting up from a sitting position because of severe pain and weakness in my legs. I was suffering severe fatigue, but thought this was due to the severe stress I had in my profession of being a deputy clerk of courts with many responsibilities, plus working a part time job.

I didn't think too much about the symptoms at the time. I didn't seek medical attention until the morning of December 1, 1972.

I had quite a surprise in store for me that morning. When I tried to get out of bed to get ready for work, I couldn't stand up or walk. My left leg and foot were contracted inwards toward my right leg and off the floor about 8 inches.

When I tried to stand on my right leg, it just gave way and I fell to the floor. After several attempts to get up, I decided. I would just crawl on my hands and knees to the telephone where I made three separate calls: one to my employer, then to my doctor who was a general practitioner at the time and then to my husband who was already at work for the day. I wanted him to go with me to the doctor as I wasn't able to get on my legs or any type of walking.

Following my doctor's appointment, I was sent to the

local hospital for many laboratory tests, X-rays, and usual tests such as routine lab work, SED rate, creatinine, etc. X-rays of my legs and back were taken to rule out any possible fractures or problems with my spine at the time.

I had these tests repeated over a course of several months without any positive findings, except for an elevated sedimentation rate. My general practitioner said in time I would probably be diagnosed with rheumatoid arthritis or Dystemic Lupus Erythromatosis.

After many periods of flares and remissions, my general practitioner felt it was advisable to send me to the Mayo Clinic in the summer of 1979.

At Mayo Clinic, I was seen by an oncologist who did my general physical examination and I had to fill out numerous documents. From the oncologist, I was sent to a Rheumatologist, who ran many laboratory tests. He told me there was nothing wrong with my blood, but if I would get into an exercise program, and go on a 1000 calorie diet to lose some weight, I just might feel somewhat better.

The Hematologist referred me to a Dermatologist as he really couldn't tell what the rash was that was covering my arms and legs. The oncologist suggested that it was possibly "shingles." When I asked the Dermatologist if he thought I had shingles, he thought not. However, the Dermatologist did help get the rash under control with some type of soaps and special creams.

From the Dermatologist, I was sent to a nutritionist, who found I had a very slow burning metabolism. She determined this through a breathing test, but she thought I could lose weight being on a 1000 calorie diet.

At this time, I was only about 30 pounds overweight and everybody was making such a big deal about my weight problem!

I am not the normal binge type eater. Actually, I don't even get "hungry." I eat because of having to take the medications.

From the nutritionist I went back to the oncologist and he said he had met with all of the physicians I had seen. They all felt that I had Osteoarthritis, obesity, Neuro-Dermatitis and Fibromyalgia.

Unfortunately, following my visit to the Mayo Clinic and using the medications they decided I should be using, my health didn't get any better.

My walking got to be increasingly worse and I still didn't lose any weight.

I saw an Orthopedic specialist at Mayo. He felt I had a rather severe curvature of my spine and ordered physical therapy treatments while I was there. They taught my husband how to do these treatments at home. This was about the best outcome of my trip to the Mayo Clinic, who are "supposedly" to be the best.

In June 1980, I suffered pulmonary embolism and following many lab tests. And, of course, X-rays again. My general practitioner said that I had a low gamma globulin count, but that he didn't want to "hang" himself on one test.

Since my health kept failing, in 1982 my GP decided to refer me to the teaching hospital not far from our hometown to see a Rheumatologist. Once again, I went through main lab tests and an exam and again told I had Fibromyalgia. Also, I needed to get into a good exercise program.

During the period of 17 years, I grew continually weaker, more fatigued, had many rashes which were always diagnosed as neurodermatitis or better known as "nerves."

Finally, in December 1989, my husband thought we should try another doctor. We transferred to another clinic in the area.

I met a young Internist who was just starting his practice. At the time, I was walking on crutches. My legs were very swollen and had a purplish rash and ulcer type lesions on them.

The first day we got to his office, he took one look at my legs and said, "I think you have Dermatomyositis." From there, I had gone to a Dermatologist, two different Neurologists, a Rheumatologist, an Endocrinologist, an Opthamologist, Orthopedist, and a surgeon.

Once again I endured many lab tests, X-rays, two EMG's, a MRI, two spinal taps and a muscle biopsy. Within six months, I was officially diagnosed with Dermatomyositis via the muscle biopsy. HURRAY!

I was finally diagnosed! No more wondering why my legs wouldn't hold me up or why the severe fatigue, or why I was having the skin problems. For the first time in 17 years, I had a diagnosis and was finally put on the proper medication.

No, my battle wasn't and isn't over. I was put on high doses of Prednisone, Plaquenil and numerous other drugs. I was on Prednisone for six years.

While most doctors don't especially care to use Prednisone for long term use because of it's many serious side effects, I really felt I needed the Prednisone for the pain. It was so severe I could hardly get any relief from any type of pain medication.

Prednisone has serious side effects and I have probably had them all, including cataracts, insulin dependent diabetes, and my upper teeth broke off at the gum line.

I have an upper plate, but these side effects were worth taking for me to get where I am today.

Here are some of the things I have to do for myself and my family while enduring this disease. I now use a draftsman's chair with wheels so I can scoot the work area in the kitchen, cooking meals and washing dishes.

I have also put my utensils I use more frequently on the lower shelves of the cupboards.

Because of the wheels on the chair, I also use it as a walker.

My husband and son were God-sends to me. I used to enjoy gardening and raising our own fruits and vegetables. They built me an "enabling garden" that I can work while on my scooter. I don't know if I'll be able to do anymore canning, but those beds will make beautiful flower beds.

My husband also built up my recliner in the family room with two blocks of 8"x8" wooden blocks. I have a special handicap chair to use in the shower, a high rise on the toilet for daytime use and a bedside commode next to the bed at night.

I use two vibrating magnetic pads with heat for my bed and the recliner. When I am in pain, I just turn on the heat and massager for 15 minutes. Oh, so much better!

How did I cope so many years with this disease? My family and I coped by continuing the search until we finally got an answer - THE DIAGNOSIS. I am blessed with very strong family support.

When anyone is ill, you find out really quick who your true friends are and you also have to believe in a Higher Power than yourself.

With Dermatomyositis, there are lots of ups and downs, flares and remissions, many hospitalizations, and sometimes newer and different symptoms.

Until a cure is found, we have to live with the disease and try to make the best of our lives for ourselves and our families.

DM Case # 7

Diagnosed 1995 - Female - Present Age 55

Five years ago, at the age of 50 (February 1995), an irritating itchy rash developed on the lower right side of my jaw. Over a period of 1.5 years, it spread to my neck, chest, back and upper thighs.

The rash across the bridge of my nose, my eyelids and cheeks were a red-purple color (later discovered to be described as *heliotrope).*

This area did not itch as much as the rest of my body. According to my Dermatologist, I was having an allergic reaction to something in Texas.

Four months prior to the initial rash, we had moved from California where I taught German and English in high school. Until this time, I had considered myself an extremely healthy woman experiencing only two C-section operations. Topical creams and a couple weeks of Prednisone didn't seem to help. The rash subsided during the winter months and became more active during the spring and summer.

The scaly rash on my chest began to peel. After several trips to the Dermatologist, he came to the conclusion that he was not dealing with a normal skin rash and suggested I might have Lupus, an autoimmune illness. He conducted his treatment and referred me to a Rheumatologist.

With the suggested diagnoses of Lupus, my husband started searching through a computer medical CD. After determining that Lupus didn't appear to be a good fit to my symptoms, he began looking for an illness that better matched my symptoms (the Internet was not as useful back during that time as it is today.)

Looking specifically for skin rash, he was surprised when he discovered a disease that had a skin rash but also had muscle weakness with difficulty swallowing as symptoms. Prior to that, we had not put together the various symptoms I had as belonging to one disease.

This one disease solved the reasons I was having difficulty swallowing, the pain and lack of strength in my legs, hips and arm muscles. The disease, of course, was Dermatomyositis (DM).

The following month involved diagnostic tests re-quested by my new doctor, a Rheumatologist. These tests included a muscle biopsy, EMG, chest x-ray, pelvic sonogram, pap smear and mammogram. The last three tests listed were to check for possibilities of cancer since I was told that 10-15% of DM patients have a malignancy causing the DM.

My CK blood test was near 400. I was so weak that I could barely get out of the bathtub. The Rheumatologist prescribed 60 mg/d Prednisone in September 1996.

The new Dermatologist (one knowledgeable about Dermatomyositis) prescribed Doxapin 10 mg, Zyrtec 10 mg/d and Triamcinoin .01% cream to be applied twice daily for the itchy rash. For six months I responded well to the medication while the Prednisone was being gradually decreased in strength.

In April 1997 my gall bladder was laparoscopically removed. It proved to be highly inflamed with numerous gall stones. No correlation between the gall bladder disease and the Dermatomyositis was indicated by the physicians.

A flare-up of the rash returned in July 1997 while I was down to 10 mg/d Prednisone. My CK was not elevated. I was introduced to 10 mg Methotrexate once a week and Folic Acid daily.

In October 1997, X-rays showed that the Prednisone was causing avascular necrosis of my hip - a good reason to lower the dosage.

Subsequently, bone density tests and X-rays showed that the tip of the fibula on both legs had been eroded, presumably by the Prednisone. Bone density was at 80% of normal!

Nevertheless, by January 1996 I was feeling great with only one itchy spot on my head.

"Feeling great" didn't last long. That same month I was diagnosed with breast cancer. A 2-CM tumor was found on one breast. It had not been detectable two months earlier by a mammogram or sonogram. The tumor was growing rapidly.

A lumpectomy quickly followed Chemotherapy and radiation were completed by September 1996. I continued with 5 mg/d Prednisone and no Methotrexate.

It was believed by most physicians that some of the drugs used in Chemotherapy would assist with the treatment of Dermatomyositis. The question remains: "Was the malignancy associated with my DM?"

For seven months I had no adverse medical problems. My hair began to grow. A flare-up of DM occurred in April 1999. At that time I was down to 3 mg/d Prednisone.

The Dermatologist pre-scribed 400 mg/d Plaquenil for the rash. At the same time, I had developed irritable bowel syndrome. In August 1999, the muscles became involved with CK at 440. The Prednisone was increased to 5 mg/d and I was put back on Methotrexate 20 mg/d. The Plaquenil was decreased to 200 mg/d.

Now it is March 2000, in a new millennium and I feel great. My CK is 162, the rash has disappeared and my muscles feel good. My strength has increased. The rash has faded. Because of the avascular narcosis, I'm unable to do impact exercises.

I do water aerobics three times a week in a nearby health center pool. I am also able to exercise on a recumbent bicycle.

The irritable bowel has improved to normal. Neither the Gastroenthrologist nor my Rheumatologist associate the bowel problem with DM. I do not agree!

It is not easy dealing with a chronic illness. The unknown future is ever present. Am I going to have another flare-up? What other side effects of the disease or the medicine might come up to bite me?

You learn to appreciate the daily experiences of life; especially, if you are having a good day. Worrying about a new hair style became insignificant when I was, instead, worried about whether my hair was going to grow back. While taking the heavy concentrations of Prednisone; later, Chemotherapy. I gained 50 pounds. Since then, I have lost 20 of them. My hair has begun to grow back and I'm looking into a new career.

You give more hugs to family and friends. During the past five years, my husband, sons, and friends have been a blessed support. I feel fortunate to have raised my boys and not be dependent upon a job for financial support. I would not repeat the past five years of my life. I am very happy to be alive!

DM Case # 8

Diagnosed 1969 - Female Present Age 30
Amy S. Trotto's Story about DM

February 10, 2000 - 29 year old female staring down her 30th birthday. My name is Amy Trotto and I cope with Dermatomyositis.

My story begins 11 years ago. I have played this story in my head thousands of times. No one to listen. No one to understand it. Back then, at 19, if you had asked me where I thought I would be at 30, I would have answered, "I am not sure if I will see my 21st birthday."

I am telling you my story today, not for your sympathy, but because I have realized there are others who need to hear this.

My story begins the summer of 1989. Approximately one month before I was to return to college for my sophomore year. I was majoring in Physical Education. It was a hot and humid August in Michigan that year. I remember it vividly, as if it were yesterday. I was working at the Garden Center as I had done since I was 16 years old. I was working many hours to earn money for school.

I had a continuing problem with an itchy rash on my hand that would come and go. I thought I was allergic to some of the plants. The next day at work, I started my search for a Dermatologist. I didn't know it would be so hard to get an appointment. I finally found one that could see me the next day. He was taking new patients.

The next day I went to the Dermatologist's office, did the preliminary paper work and waited to be called. When they called me in, the Dermatologist asked me of my problem and looked at my hands. I also mentioned there was some itching on my knees, a little on my face, but the bumps on my hands couldn't be seen.

I told the doctor that I worked with plants and chemicals and out in the sun most of the day. He immediately called in his partner.

They both inspected my hands, asking me some strange questions regarding if I had been sick recently, allergies, muscle weakness, etc. I denied every thing. I was tired, but I was working 50-60 hours a week in the sun. They said that might be the problem, but they wanted to see me in two weeks.

I left with some ointment, told to wear sun screen with the highest SPF.

A week and half before leaving for school, my second appointment with Dr. Mopple came. I told him the rash was still there and I was feeling out of shape.

Immediately they started with words I didn't know: Collagen disease and Lupus. They began scheduled blood work and called a Rheumatologist, had an EMG, and was transferred to the University of Michigan. The doctors thought I had Dermatomyositis; a week later a biopsy was scheduled. No one explained anything.

The day I had the biopsy, I began Prednisone 60 mg/d.

I took the first pill on the first day of school; immediately sick at my stomach. I called the doctor - and three days later he returned the call.

After the biopsy, I was seen at the hospital weekly which wasn't easy. I did not have a car and I was two hours away at school, caring a full load and had a job.

At the first appointment, I had to wait three hours before seeing me for about 10 minutes. The doctors consulted among themselves for two hours, excluding me.

When they returned, I had to have more blood work - I was scared to death of needles!! Then the lab technician complained it being closing time, so she wasn't happy about taking 10 vials of blood.

Within a month of beginning Prednisone, I couldn't sleep; my heart beat was racing at top speed. Soon my face turned to "moon face," my stomach had swollen until it appeared as if I were pregnant.

I hated getting up each morning to face myself in the mirror. The black circles around my eyes because of lack of sleep looked so bad that I knew my room mates and others were staring at me.

The second appointment at the hospital didn't go any better. I was basically ignored, given something - Restori - to let me sleep.

I began having extreme pain in both knees, scaring me, and I called home at 4:00 A.M.

Two days later the hospital returned my call. I explained to the Rheumatologist the situation. He put me on an anti-inflammatory medicine and Zantac for my stomach. My knees wouldn't allow me to squat or climb steps. My knees looked as big as cantaloupes. The doctor drained my knees, removing much fluid which helped.

Prior to Christmas, my sleeping problems were over, but I couldn't get out of bed, no motivation, extremely paranoid, and depressed. I looked like a freak.

When I became afraid of people, panic attacks began; my memory became blurred; then my parents thought I had become suicidal (I wasn't).

The day after Christ- mas, I was in a terrible mental condition. The doctor was on vacation but I got an appointment with his substitute. He was extremely rude, wanting to send me to a mental hospital.

My mother got an appointment with a psychiatrist and after answering many questions, he told me to return to my doctor telling him the psychiatrist had found a massive infection. After seeing the disgruntled doctor, he said I needed to go to the hospital; but changed his mind after speaking with the psychiatrist, giving a prescription for antibiotics and sent me home. I was confused, lay on the sofa for the next week; everything making me cry.

Having a hard time, sad and lonely, back in school I couldn't concentrate. I decided to quit school since I couldn't do all the physical things required for the Physical Education program.

PRESENT: I began to rebuild my life; had a chance to start over and to learn about my disabilities. There have been rough times.

Currently, I have a good marriage, a good job and lots of friends. I don't think about the Dermatomyositis all time like I once did.

I feel very grateful to be able to move on with my life. I hope everyone with the disease has learned to cope mentally and physically and may go into remission as I have done.

DM Case # 9

Female

What I think has gotten me through Dermatomyositis are through grace, grit, the prayers of people all over the world (thanks to my music) and the songs I've written during some very bad times during the flare-ups of Dermatomyositis

I had near death experiences because of respiratory muscle weakness and the errors of doctors.

Probably the best thing that happened was a six month time of horrible complications of hysterectomy while on Chemo. The surgeons - best on the East Coast - the opportunity to get to all the anger of my lifetime in one full swoop.

I had three major surgeries, two minor CT-abscess drainage procedures, 2.5 months of PICC line with multiple antibiotics, finally culminating with an obstructed intestine.

After going through all this, Dermatomyositis seemed easy. At the end of that ordeal, I didn't have any energy left to have any anger and the original, arrogant surgeon was so happy I wasn't going to sue him.

I am so happy to be alive and have learned how to be "present" with my doctors so they see me as a person rather than a person with a disease. We work together as a team to fight this Myositis.

The near death experienced arose from the sleep apnea and are stories within themselves. Some of the songs I've written come whole and complete during severe apnea times. It is good to see how these songs touch other people.

The worst part of DM is the isolation I feel when I'm sick; dealing with fair weather friends who disappear until I'm well again. When I am better and able to perform, the phone rings off the hook. I don't bother with fair weather friends; it's their loss, not mine. I have my own life to live.

The disease is very, very hard on my husband and 12-year old son. My Rheumatologist, though, is a wonderful woman, tells me my son will grow up to be stronger, more compassionate and understanding because of my DM conditions. I sure hope so!!

Well, this started out as a short message, but I keep going on and on.

I've found that pre-tending is a big help to me. In other words, if I want to walk out to the barn in the back, or pull weeds from the garden, I just pretend it is something I do every day and, sometimes, I surprise myself!

You've heard the saying, if you can only wiggle a toe, then wiggle that toe; and in a while you might be able to wiggle more than one toe.

DM Case # 10

Diagnosed 1996 - Female
Present Age 44

My birth name is Cathie. I am 44 years old who has been enduring Dermatomyositis. I consider myself to be 70% recovered and very lucky.

My blood work is now normal, including my SED rate which was at 37, now is 11. My LDH was 973, now is 181. Manual muscle strength test score was 2 (O being paralyzed and 5 being normal), now at 5 with the exception of a 4.5 right hip flexor. My trunk muscles were badly damaged. I could barely lift my head, now I am able to do three full sit ups. My ANA is still positive with a speckled pattern titre of 1:640.

Here are some things I've learned while having DM:

Hope is everything.

Energy is a precious gift to be spent wisely.

Disease brings us to our knees to give us a different view on life and what is really important.

The body can heal itself if you feed and take care of it.

Listen to your body.

Nurture your soul by being creative during your rest periods. Read, write, paint, doodle or medicate.

Love your self like you were your own best friend.

Read up on your illness and medications. Knowledge is powerful.

Doctor shop: Don't stop searching until you find the doctor you feel comfortable with.

Use your doctor as a resource/aide, not a cure. Challenge them if you are in question and ask them questions.

A person with a chronic illness needs support. Join a support group and become active in it.

My primary illness is DM. I also suffer from other secondary illnesses: clinical depression, Sjogens, Fibromyalgia, and Raynauds.

DM is a connective tissue disease, that if left alone, untreated, could possibly bring death 3 to 5 years. Inflammation occurs in the joints, muscles and sometimes the organs.

The main areas that are affected are the shoulder and hip girdle and the throat. Having weakened hip girdle muscles creates difficulty in getting up or sitting down or using steps.

The weak shoulder muscles cause difficulty in lifting, putting on a heavy coat, or holding up your arms to comb your hair.

When the throat is affected, you frequently feel a choking sensation and have a problem swallowing. The skin develops a rash that is red, splotchy and very itchy. Fatigue is a big problem and sometimes you can only do one thing a day because you are so weak.

MEDICAL HISTORY: I went into a severe clinical depression in August 1994. A year later, I fell from a ladder, landing on my hip and hand. Immediately I began to suffer from symptoms of Fibromyalgia and it was difficult to do physical activities.

In December 1995, I collapsed and had to quit work as an Event Coordinator. In February 1996, the doctor noticed my muscles were falling away from the bones.

I began the medical testing: blood and urine tests, EMG, and a muscle biopsy, being diagnosed with DM in April 1996.

MEDICATIONS: Starting with Methotrexate until March 1997, quitting cold turkey.

Currently I am taking Doxycycline 200 mg/d and Intravenous Clindamycain 900 mg and began taking many other alternative medicines.

(Editor's note: The writer gives several pages of her experiences with the drugs, her diet, body massages of several types, and her methods of exercises and stretching. Space does not allow.)

What I experienced the year I was on traditional treatment:

Although these treatments and medications helped with

reducing the inflammation and clearing the rash, I went into a clinical depression and other problems.

After stop taking all these medications and treatments, everything returned to normal except for the weight gain.

(Editor's note: We had to delete several pages detailing 12 months. month by month of some of the good and the bad times and bad experiences.)

I would like to share with you my current status.

EMOTIONAL HEALTH:

I believe that depression has an organic cause and if the physical problem is addressed, the emotional problems will improve. Now that DM is under control, the depression is gone, and I once again enjoy a happy, social life.

I surround myself with loving, nurturing people and have given up my old life style.

PHYSICAL HEALTH: I am physically active and accomplish many daily activities. My energy level has increased dramatically. I am able to enjoy the gym, swimming, walking, dancing, cooking and travel.

My rash only remains on my hand and my muscle tone is slowly returning to normal. The Fibromyalgia symptoms have improved considerably. I am ready to start doing some volunteer work outside my home, which I hope will lead me eventually back into the work force and financial independence.

I have started a support group at a hospital in Manitoba, Canada for those interested. Spreading hope to others is my passion. I consider it an honor to have this purpose.

We all hope a cure is just around the corner, but until then, we use the therapy as a kinder and gentler substitute.

(Editors note: Please check with your personal physician before you attempt any methods and medicines. We do not advocate any particular method of treatment of Myositis.)

DM Case # 11

Diagnosed 1984
Female - Present Age 56

In 1984, age 41, I became very ill. I was unable to walk or take care of my personal needs alone. I was very sore, weak, running a high temperature, and in severe pain.

I was hospitalized and after seven days of testing, my Rheumatologist diagnosed my disease as Dermatomyositis and began treating it with 80 mg/d of Prednisone. The Prednisone was like a miracle drug for me: I didn't realize, though, what a long hard road I had ahead of me.

All my major muscles have been destroyed by the disease and I was started on physical therapy. There was a very long recovery period. I never realized just how this rare disease called Dermatomyositis would change my life. I had two children - a son, 21 years old, and a 15-year old daughter, both living at home. This was a very difficult time for them.

For years after I was diagnosed, I felt my husband was uncaring and unloving toward me. This was very hard on my recovery and the progression of my disease. I suffered a lot of hurt and pain during that very difficult time of my life.

Thanks to very wonderful parents and a sister who helped take very good care of me, I am still around today.

I have spent many days in loneliness and complete solitude. I don't think I was ever sad. I must say, however, for the last several years my husband has been wonderful. Now I actually feel loved.

My life has changed in so many ways. I can't do most of the things I did before I got this disease. I can't take care of my home like I did before, and this has been one of the hardest things I've had to accept. I now realize there's more to life than a perfect home.

I have learned a lot about what is important in life, and it is not things. Now, I try to do what I can to help other people and I like to send lots of cards to people. If I can make someone else's day better, I feel better about myself.

Now, I am 56 years old, living and coping with a severe case of Dermatomyositis. During the last 16 years I have been hospitalized 14 times. I was hospitalized with pulmonary thrombosis and fibrosis in both lungs, and while there, developed pneumonia in both lungs.

Several months later, I was treated with Methotrexate, which caused me to develop shingles and I had to be hospitalized again. I've been given Methotrexate several times since then for short periods. I've taken Imuran and Plaquenil, which didn't seem to help me.

My doctor also treated me with IVIg - immunoglobulin . He didn't seem to think it helped me much and it was very expensive. I would like to try it again.

I've never been completely taken off Prednisone since my disease has never be in remission. At this time, I'm taking 40 mg of Prednisone every other day. Because of the Prednisone, I've developed cataracts, diabetes, high blood pressure and osteoporosis. The osteoporosis caused a compression fracture in my lower spine. I have acute Calcinosis, which has caused a lot of suffering. I feel like my body is full of rocks. I can't lie or sit comfortably.

My Calcinosis has resulted in two very large tumors, one in each thigh. In 1992, I had surgery to remove a tumor from my right thigh. I hemorrhaged, and I required five major surgeries in one week. These surgeries about resulted in my death. While hospitalized, I got the flu and pneumonia in both lungs. Later, I had two more surgeries to deride the wound. I almost lost my leg. It took two years for my wound to heal.

Four years later, I had a second operation to remove a calcium tumor in my left thigh. My Rheumatologist and surgeon sent me to the University of Pittsburgh Hospital. Before I left, the tumor had ruptured and was severely infected and gangrened. My doctors here weren't sure the doctors in Pittsburgh could help me, but they were my last hope.

After a six hour ambulance ride, I arrived at the University of Pittsburgh Hospital. I was started on very high doses of antibiotics. A team of doctors decided they could do the surgery, which lasted 5.5 hours.

They removed a large chunk of calcium and one of my hamstring muscles. During the surgery, an orthopedic surgeon removed what calcium he could from around my sciatic nerve. He could not remove it from the nerve itself.

Later, I had to have another surgery to deride the wound. I still don't have good feelings in my leg. So, thanks to a very wonderful team of doctors, I survived the operation and was on my way to a long and hard recovery.

After arriving back home, I had home care nurses for four months. My surgeon here helped care for my leg. I decided after all the suffering not to have a skin graft. It took one year for the wound to heal. Thanks to excellent doctors and nurses, and very good care, my leg and my life were saved.

In early 1999, I again became very ill. I did not want to eat anything. I was hospitalized and was told that my potassium was very low and I had anorexia.

My heart was beating irregularly and I was very weak and very nauseous. My PCP gave me potassium in every known form and the next morning, it was gone.

She finally found that my kidneys were dumping my potassium and started me on 25 mg/d of Spironolactone. It has helped so far.

My Gastrologist found my stomach did not empty completely and put me on 80 mg/d of Propulsid. Recently, it was revealed that Propulsid is a very dangerous drugs, so I am now taking Raglan.

My eating problem had become so bad and I had suffered so much that I did not want to live. I was nauseous all my waking hours. All I thought about was how much I didn't want to eat, but I have to eat. I did not want to wake up in the mornings because I knew I had to eat. I had to force myself to eat. I knew I was losing the battle.

Finally, my PCP called in a group of mental health experts and very quickly they diagnosed me with depression. I must admit that I was suicidal. They started me on medication and I'm doing much better now. I still worry about it happening again. If it does, I don't know how I could go on. That really scares me.

My disease also caused me to have hemolytic anemia from which I nearly died. Initially, I was treated with 800 mg of IV Prenisolone and then very high does of Prednisone, reducing as necessary. So far, my Hematologist has kept it under control.

Summer is a very difficult time for me because of my Calcinosis. It really bothers me that I can't wear short sleeves or shorts. However, I enjoy getting outside and taking short trips. The sun is also a very big problem for me. As much as I can, I try to stay out of direct sunlight, wear lotion, sunglasses and a hat. I even have to be careful not to get too much exposure in the sun while riding in a car.

I'm thankful to be here. Every day I thank God for being so good to me and blessing me with so much. He is my Strength. *("I can do all things through Christ which strengtheneth me. - Philippians 4:13)*

I now have five beautiful grandchildren who are such a joy to me and help me make it through each day.
I pray that in some way
I can touch each of their lives and make them better people. Not only has my Derma-tomyositis been a great teacher for me, I feel that is has also been one for the grandchildren. Already at their tender ages, they are so kind and thoughtful. They keep me going.

I know I have many more changes coming in my life. My goal is to enjoy life more. I especially would like to help others with Dermatomyositis. I would like to say to those who have this disease, "Don't give you." God bless you all.

DM Case # 12

Diagnosed Aug. 1999
Female Hispanic - Present Age 47

I am a 47 year old Hispanic female, Navy retiree and I was recently diagnosed with DM (August and September, 1999). Prior to this fate, I was always very athletic - constantly involved in a variety of sports - volleyball, racquet ball, bowling, jogging 5-to-10 miles daily, and I had begun bike riding and swimming.

I was losing weight and feeling great! My doctor even took me off of Glucotrol (my second type of diabetes medication) and my sugar levels were within normal standards.

The following symptoms appeared over night in August 1999. I had all the symptoms: butterfly shaped rash on chest, arms - constant itching/burning - and the rash was beginning to show up on my face; and almost total loss of strength in all my muscles.

I could not lift my arms without them aching and I couldn't lift myself out of a chair without my leg muscles hurting. I had to be turned over in bed because my muscles had little or no strength with lots of pains, feeling like pins and needles

My CPK level was over 2000. I had to lean on my elbows to brush my teeth. I couldn't dress myself or even brush my hair. The Sunday prior to admittance into the hospital, I awoke with a throbbing in my right eye. My husband looked at me and from the look on his face, I had to question him.

I looked in the mirror to see my whole right side of my face swollen so much had almost closed my eye. This was truly a scary situation for me.

Being a diabetic (type ll) daily medication: Glugophase 2000, Prednisone 10 mg and Methotrexate 25 mg/weekly. From August to September 1999, I had to undergo several tests to confirm the disease. I had to have several EMGs, various blood work and a muscle biopsy. After my diagnosis was confirmed in September 1999, I was hospitalized with 1000 mg Prednisone IV. A colonoscopy checked for any tumor, then was given Methotrexate on my third day in the hospital.

Since then I have been on Methotrexate, steroids, pain pills, a Glugophase (diabetic medicine). So far, so good. Everyday I see a marked improvement. I am able to walk longer hours with little pain. My medications do have some side effects (nausea, diarrhea) but at least I am not suffering like I was seven months ago.

My job has been very supportive of my disease. I was

placed on short-term disability.

During the six months I was home, I attempted to take short distance walks (about a block), just to build up my energy, but at times I found that I would get a shortness of breath. During these times I cut my walks to a much shorter distance. I was determined to keep busy as much as I could.

The more I kept myself busy, the less likelihood of depression regarding the disease. Until I was diagnosed with DM, I had no idea how many muscles are affected throughout the body. It has no limitations regarding it's pain level.

One minute I could be fine, with only a small amount of pain, but bearable, and then the next, it would slap me down with a jolt.

January, March and April I had blood work performed and the results were outstanding. My CPK levels were within normal ranges (40 or less). My concern is the fact there isn't enough research performed regarding DM.

There are several theories, but no known cures, only treatments. I was taught how to inject myself with the Methotrexate and that in itself was emotionally involved.

Effective in February 2000, I was authorized to return to work. I am an office manager and perform computer work eight hours daily. I have attempted to work at least 40 hours a week, but some weeks I am only able to perform 32 hours.

Prior to DM, I worked an average of 60 hours weekly. I have had to undergo various life style changes as well due to DM.

I can no longer even attempt to perform any of my sports activities. Housework is sometimes difficult to do.

But I do have one consolidation: my family. My family has been very supportive of my needs. My biggest enemy has been myself - stubbornness. I have a tendency to "forget" I have DM and do things I shouldn't be doing, such as yard work.

I have always been very athletic and enthusiastic. I find these are difficult to achieve these days.

My spirits are high. So is my sense of humor. Since I was told of Dermatomyositis, I have researched throughout the Internet and have located several web sites and have made new friends.

I have attempted to spread my sense of humor and high spirits to others; who like me, have had their share of trying days. I only hope and pray that one day technology will find a cure for DM, PM, IBM, and JDM.
- Vickie Vinson

DM Case # 13

Female - Present Age 36

January 11, 1995
The Day that Changed My Life

I had decided to return to school. My husband and I were building our home and everything seemed to be going great in my life at 31 years of age. My husband and I were wanting to have children and felt the time was getting right for us to start a family.

But a problem arose. I began to tire easily, my muscles were extremely sore and felt like I had bruising that was not visible to the eye. I literally would lay down in the afternoon, no matter where I was and fall asleep for a solid two or more hours.

My husband massaged Aspercream on my shoulders nightly. I lived on Advil all day to help control the pain. My hands had developed a stiffening soreness too.

Bill, my husband, was worried about me and asked that I see a doctor. Me? Sick, never! The only sickness I had were childhood illnesses, but nothing as an adult.

I had never been to a doctor except to my Gynecologist. My stepfather is a physician and I mentioned my symptoms to him without any worry from him. But to appease my husband, I made an appointment with the Gynecologist.

I told her of my ailments, sore muscles, stiff and swollen fingers, a rash inside my eye; how easily I tired, that my jaw had begun popping. When asked what I thought might be the cause. I laughed and said "old age?" She laughed as I had just turned 31 years of age.

She ordered numerous tests for me. I wasn't worried, the thought of me being really sick was hard to imagine.

The weekend after the appointment, Bill and I went out of town for a long weekend. Upon returning, there was a phone message from the Gynecologist telling me she had scheduled an appointment for me to see Dr. Morgan, an internal specialist.

This sent the red flag up for me! I called my parents and asked what could be going on. My stepfather called my Gynecologist, calling back to say everything was under control and not to worry.

My mother and sister went with me to see Dr. Morgan. I must have still been in denial that there couldn't possibly be anything really wrong with me.

Dr. Morgan talked with me awhile. He had all my lab work from the Gynecologist. He diag-nosed me with Dermatomyositis.

I didn't have a clue what he was talking about. I couldn't even say the word so he wrote it down for me on paper. He explained a bit about the disease and left to get literature about DM for me. I walked into the waiting room, called my sister and Mom to the exam room. I literally couldn't speak when they asked what was the diagnosis. I pointed to the word on the paper: "Dermatomyositis."

Dr. Morgan returned with the literature and explained the disease to my Mom and sister. I don't remember a thing he said.

Mom and my sister Kelly went to eat lunch. I called my step-dad from the restaurant to let him know the diagnosis. Then I called my husband and told him about the appointment. We had a quiet lunch. None of us talked. They realized the magnitude of what I had been diagnosed with.

I stopped by my husband's office. He was really upset. Another doctor's office had called him to schedule a muscle biopsy date for me. I was to have the biopsy the next morning. I just couldn't believe what was happening.

The biopsy confirmed the diagnosis. I was then scheduled to see a doctor in Dallas, a drive of about 4.5 hours from our home. Dr. Morgan felt the Dallas doctors would have more experience with Dermatomyositis. I was sent to see a Rheumatologist.

The next week Bill and I drove to Dallas and the following week. Eventually we returned to Dallas every 4-to-6 weeks to see the doctor. In the meantime, I had started on Prednisone. The Rheumamatologist assured me the disease would be in remission in about a year. Unfortunately, that was over five years ago and many trips ago. I have never been in remission.

I began searching the Internet for Myositis patients, but found none. I felt so alone with this disease; no one to talk with or to relate with who would know my feelings. My family didn't have a clue about the disease.

I bloated because of Prednisone and felt miserable. After six months, I began to take the pill form of Methotrexate. After ten months on Prednisone, I couldn't think straight, my arms felt like a ton of concrete. I felt suicidal and just plain crazy.

Dr. Morgan started me on Zoloff. After ten days on the medication, the cloud lifted and I returned to my old happy self again. It was unbelievable the difference I felt mentally. I was taking 800 mg of calcium daily since the Prednisone was so terrible for my bones.

A year and half after the diagnosis, I stopped taking the Methotrexate because of the mouth ulcers it caused. The Prednisone was increased and decreased for another year. I began to take Methotrexate again along with a prescription for Folic Acid to counteract the side effects. This seemed to help a bit.

I began having severe hip problems and could not walk without pain. I have a high pain tolerance, but the pain was so severe I stayed in bed. X-rays and bone density scans didn't show any abnormalities. Thank-fully, the pain subsided on its own.

A month shy of the four years after diagnosis, I began taking Methotrexate by shots. My digestive system could no longer digest the Methotrexate by pills.

During these years I had constantly been on Prednisone,

taking the 800 mg calcium daily and a squirt of Miacalcin into my nose; also taking the Folic Acid and multivitamins.

Four years after diagnosis, I began taking Cyclosporine. Now that was a killer medication! I never had been so sick! Fevers, night sweats, nightmares, felt horrible! Getting out of bed was a huge effort. After 11 months on this medication, I began falling and hurting myself. I discontinued the Cyclosporine and felt so much better immediately.

Later, I went to see a doctor in Tulsa, Oklahoma. He prescribed I-Carnitine and Riboflavin vitamins to help rebuild the muscles.

I learned DM has several stages and the doctor didn't know which stage I was in. That was eight weeks ago and I have not heard a word from that doctor.

I began feeling that all the trips to Dallas to see the Rheumatologist and the toxic medications had shown no significant change with the disease.

I was fed up with fighting the disease the doctor's way. I began fighting DM my own way.

After five years and two months, I stopped taking Methotrexate. Five weeks after that, I discontinued the Prednisone and took absolutely no other medications. I never told the Tulsa or Dallas doctors as they didn't have a clue how horrible the medications made me feel.

I started hurting now that the medications were out of my system. I had watched a TV story about a healer from the UK that comes to the U.S. to help those who wanted to see her. She comes to the States twice a year: I missed both chances of seeing her.

Luckily, I found a healer in the city where we live. She taught me how to meditate and has done an inner session on me, removing the pain. It worked!!

I was pain-free and able to sleep through the night after the intercession. I meditate daily and she meditates daily for me.

Another intercession is scheduled this week. I am so excited! I feel as though God led me to this wonderful lady with this special gift!

I began an exercise routine and I walk nightly. I need to

rebuild the muscle I lost over the past five years and four months.

Things are looking great for me. I am now 36 years old, turning 37 this year. Hopefully, we will finally be able to start our family in the near future.

There is one statement to this day I hate to hear after being asking how I feel. If I truthfully had told how I felt, which 9 out of 10 times was horrible, the response from the questioner would be, "Well, you look great."

Please remember DM and the other Myositis diseases are not attacking us outwardly, but it is doing it's damage inwardly.

I believe Lisa Mailhes with the Lupus Foundation said it best, "People may look great from the outside, but that's not always the case."

If anyone would like to contact me, please do so at karen-Myositis@hotmail.com.

DM Case # 14

Diagnosed Feb. 1996
Female - Present Age 65

I hope my story fits within the guidelines for the book.

At first, I didn't think I needed to state that I was female; my name would be enough. Then I remembered another Alouise at one of our MAA Conferences. HE was from Germany.

Illness is never funny, but I have had funny things happen to and I have had wonderful people to help along the way. Humor is a way I cope.

I had to hand write this. My left wrist had carpal tunnel surgery on Monday. The computer taunts me when I press the wrong button and everything falls to the floor or goes to the ceiling.
- Alouise Ritter, Hartfield, Virginia

The discomfort of Dermatomyositis is like having a family of sleeping hedgehogs (*picture of a 'hedgehog' was enclosed)* inside the muscles. When one of those little guys shifts, a pain-burn-itch goes to the surface of the skin from deep down inside and requires immediate attention.

First, I massage the area. If that doesn't work, I apply a lotion or ice or bag balm. If none of these relieve, I shower to cool the skin and then apply lotion.

I was diagnosed with DM in February, 1996 when I was 61 years old. The Urgent Care staff at Leigh Hospital in Norfolk, Virginia took aggressive action when they suspected DM or Lupus.

Blood work was done immediately. Prednisone was prescribed and I was sent to a Rheumatologist and Dermatologist the next day.

The Rheumatologist added Methotrexate to my medication therapy. The combination caused stress to my digestive system. My mouth was lined with sores and I would wake up at night crying with severe pain in my esophagus. A container of vanilla Yoplat Yogurt would comfort.

I am taking Metho-trexate by injection which relieved some of the side effects mentioned.

The Dermatologist took a muscle biopsy and referred me for a MRI. These procedures confirmed I had Dermatomyositis.

Plaquenil was added to my medicines. This caused more rash and itching.

Imuran was given in place of Plaquenil. This caused more distress to the skin and stomach.

DM seemed to attack me very suddenly. I awakened one morning unable to comb my hair and had to have help dressing. A box was used to raise my dinner plate closer to my mouth. I could feed myself.

After four years, it is still difficult for me to open my mouth wide enough to eat a hamburger and bun; just hamburger and half the bun will suffice.

I was too weak to lift pots and pans and do household tasks. It was six months or more before I could resume driving and other activities.

Because muscles are weak, falling is a given. One of my classic stories took place during a morning walk with my husband.

I fell in front of a tavern (I choose to get myself up because I know where I hurt). I returned to an upright position and continued the walk.

An ambulance appeared. Should I "run" back and lay down on the sidewalk? The EMT's realized I was the victim and gave me an ice pack for my badly bruised hand.

Physical Therapy is ESSENTIAL. Rest is ESSENTIAL.

More recently I fell and broke my ankle. Therapy helped regain strength and balance. Now I'm more consistent with exercise at the Fitness Center. Daily walking is not good enough to reach various muscles needing help.

DM will go into remission but not for long. Skin flairs are painful. Even a hug will cause a body to cringe. Snuggling with my beloved becomes unbearable. Without a caring husband and family, this would be a lonely, devastating illness.

My Dermatologist re-commends as many as two showers daily, enough to moisten the body and before the body dries, apply a lotion bought over the counter: (1) Cetaphel (2) Bag Balm.

Lotions prescribed: (1) Triamcinoline Acetonide Creme 0.1%; (2) Betamechasone Sarna Silver Sulfadiazine Creme was prescribed for skin ulcers. For best results, cover without a bandage.

I wear loose fitting cotton/cotton blend clothes. Because my arms are badly marred, I wear jackets or other long sleeved garments when I am away from home. Slacks or other garments which are tight are only worn when working out at the Fitness Center.

Presently, I am mobile, able to drive and do most of the things I enjoyed before my illness. I have to rest more.

Some days are worse and then for some unknown reason, a good day or several, will permit activities requiring energy.

There are publications which suggest removing wheat flour from the diet. I have been using spelt or rice flour breads and pastas for eight weeks. Time will tell if this is beneficial. I am better. Why? I don't know.

Medications taken since February 1996:

* *means I'm now taking.*

Prednisone - good for short period of time.

* Methotrexate - needed for muscles; seldom helps skin.

* Folic Acid - maintains good liver and no side effects.

Leucover - bad side effects, stomach upset

Prozac - good in early stages of illness.

Imuran - prescribed three times; bad side effects.

* Prilosec - controls reflux

* Ambien - needed for sleep.

Atarax - prescribed to stop itching; didn't work.

* Celebrix - *Sometimes* relieves inflammation skin.

Dapsome - bad side effects; caused ulcers and burns on skins.

DM is inconsistent. Sometimes a lotion or medication will work one time and not another. There seems to be no set of rules on how to deal with Dermatomyositis.

- Alouise W. Ritter Hartfield, Virginia

DM Case # 15

Diagnosed 1998
Female - Present Age 35

My name is Donna Bueche and I live in Illinois, in a northern suburb of Chicago. I am 35 years old, married 14 years and am a stay-at-home mom of two young boys. I went to college for one year and I did office temporary work before having children. I have had Dermatomyositis for two years. I am considered to be going into remission and now tapering medications (Prednisone and Methotrexate).

Some days I cope with my Myositis disease better than others. On good days, I have a strong, fighting attitude.. That is because remissions seems to be imminent. My CPK levels have come down and stabilized and I am allowed to exercise now.

I take much less pain medication now. (Antiflammatories: my doctor will not give me narcotics. For this, I usually praise his wisdom and responsibility. At other times, I curse him for it.)

On a bad day, I do not cope as well. When I have pain, weakness, fatigue and depression, my obligations and responsibilities (which, I have learned to keep to a minimal) seem as if they are piled too high. Those are the days when I reach the end of my rage and I have to tie a knot and just hang on and wait - because things always change!

To me, coping and healing have meant drawing upon every resource I can think of and to continually re-shuffle, re-evaluate and re-prioritize according to my options.

I have definitely had to learn to "go with the flow" to give up control of many things to still strive and be happy amid chaos.

I have learned to retain hope when living a nightmare; to endure a hellish situation; to embrace life once again, even when life has "let me down" so profoundly; to trust the degree of health I have, even knowing how fragile and precarious it can become; and to choose to grow wise and loving instead of bitter and resentful. (Again, I say, some days are better than others!)

I am a better person for what I have been through. This is not to say that a person needs to get sick to gain wisdom or make spiritual strides such as I have made, because they certainly do not. But this is the way it has been with me.

For example, I now have empathy for the sick and disabled. I thought I did before, because I was polite, but really, I didn't.

I was merely con-descending. I did not know it was like this. I was judgmental. I did not know I was like this before. I have now walked a mile in their shoes, so to speak. I now really know that a human being sits in a wheelchair and now I can look them in the eye.

It is so important to have a competent specialist (Rheumatologist or Neurologist) you trust and to do what he prescribes.

I am very fortunate to have an intelligent and intuitive Rheumatologist who cares. When he told me to begin Methotrexate, and chemotherapy drugs, I did not want to do it. I was afraid I was putting poison into my body.

And I wasn't thrilled about taking Prednisone either. I finally realized that it is okay to receive the drugs as healing energy. For this, the medicine is a gift.

I held the pills in my hands and prayed they would do only good and nothing bad to my body. The goal of the Methotrexate therapy is to suppress the immune system enough to calm down the autoimmune activity, but not too much.

My doctor told me he wanted to see my white blood cell count reduced by half. Because the white blood cells were attacking my skin and skeletal muscles. I would visualize this cell activity and reduction taking place.

I would visualize the remaining blood cells were still available and strong and doing their proper jobs within my immune system. I prayed for minimal side effects, especially not to lose my hair. I believe in the power of prayer and I believe my prayers were specifically answered.

I would like to offer hope to anyone diagnosed with DM. It can get better with drug therapy. Work really hard by keeping your doctor appointments. Cultivate patience, because it will probably take some time to see measurable results. Take all the little pills. Try to endure the side effects. Read and learn all you can. Pray. If it has been awhile, or if you never have prayed, now is a good time to start. I pray to my Lord and Savior, Jesus Christ.

If you improve enough like I have, you get to go to physical therapy. I put off making any first appointment for two months because I thought I couldn't fit it into my schedule.

I thought there were more important priorities in my and my families' lives. My doctor finally made me realize it was important to go to physical therapy and I have been going for a few weeks now and I am just ecstatic to be exercising and building my strength again. But it is slow going.

You do not bounce back from this. I am shocked at the

amount of weakness and damage that was done during my bout with DM. It is scary to face. My left leg is much weaker than my right. But on the day after physical therapy, I take much less pain medication and I feel so energetic; almost normal again.

Another way I cope is that I began a home-based business doing something I love (selling collectibles on the Internet.) I highly recommend if you are sick with a chronic illness, find something new or perhaps something long abandoned that you are compassionate about and do it. Sometimes when you are absorbed in concentration and lose track of time: something you love so much that you will push through the pain to do it anyway (with doctor approval, of course.) Don't be afraid to start something new and daring. Don't worry what will happen if your disease worsens. Go for it anyway. Your passion may just enhance your healing. Tomorrow will come anyway and tomorrow will take care of itself.

It is hard to remember how I got through the worse part of my illness, about six months ago, when my pain and weakness peaked. I coped very differently then because all I could do was to survive.

I was in so much pain and there were so many tests and procedures. Many, many blood draws, a MRI, an EMG and a muscle biopsy. I am so glad the bulk of the tests and procedures are over for the present time.

I have moved from blood work every three weeks to a three-month schedule. I remember when I was at my sickest, that I was barely able to walk with my first-grader to his bus stop.

Yet, I was so grateful that I could do it. I had my infant to care for and we moved twice. I do not know how I got through this. I found out how strong a person has to be when absolutely necessary. We can keep on going long after we think we can't go another step. When you are very sick for a long time, you must get this out for yourself!

During that time, I read good books by Bernie Siegal and Steven Levine. I read everything at the websites and I participated on the message boards at those sites, talking with others who have a Myositis disease or who have a child with one. Those message boards were my lifeline for awhile. Since we have a rare disease, there is not a Myositis support group on every corner. In this regard, the Internet really helps. You can find support for everything from practical to emotional issues that are unique to us. Like that Cetaphel liquid soap is great for our hands; that muscle twitching is completely normal for DM patients even though it never seems to be listed as a symptom anywhere.

I believe as long as you are drawing breath, there is hope and reason to go on. (And I know that breathing itself can become a challenge when you have DM.) Gifts come. You can change wonderfully for the better with greater depth of character.

For instance, I used to wonder why some people were so crabby and miserable in public. Now I know that maybe they are not feeling well. Maybe they do not feel well at all, but they still have to be out buying groceries, etc.

Or how that I used to look down my nose at a mom in public with dirty hair and unkempt, badly behaved children. Now I realize that this woman may be in Chemotherapy for all anyone knows and has an energy level of zero.

Of when I used to see an overweight person in a wheelchair or on one of those motorized carts at the store. I realize they may be bloated from inactivity that is not of their choosing, and/or a high Prednisone dose that is required to save their life

I know there are many people who have true empathy and compassion for the sick and disabled and they did not have to get sick or have a loved one get sick to learn about it. I admire that and stand in awe of them. I did not learn it until I got sick. Really sick.

I am not implying that I got sick because I need to learn these lessons or be punished. I do not believe it works that way. I am just explaining how I found a lesson and a gift for myself and made some good come from a bad situation.

Frankly, I sometimes feel that I have learned enough lessons and have done enough character building for a lifetime!

My next goal for myself is to consistently look my best

when I appear in public. How I miss that! How I would enjoy this return to an aspect of my former self. But I am forever changed!. If I go out looking like a million bucks, I am not proud or haughty. I thank the Lord I had the strength and ability to comb my own hair.

Living with chronic illness is not like the movies where people have perfect problems. Managing a chronic illness is grueling, grungy, ungraceful work. It shows what you are made of, right down to your core.

If you don't like everything you find there, it is learning to forgive yourself. It is picking yourself up over and over again, many times alone. It is worth it.

I take one of the new class of antidepressant drugs and I know I would not be faring as well without it. The antidepressant helps to keep me focused and thinking with the right mind so that I am able to "pull myself up by my bootstraps" and carry on.

It is our responsibility to ask clearly and specifically for the things we need from friends, family and loved ones. They cannot read our minds. They have lives with energy-sapping problems of their own. But people like to help.

My friends, family and loved ones would do anything for me. I know I do not utilize this resource enough. I don't ask them and I try to do everything I can myself. I have refused offers of help. I like to be in control and to be the one giving and helping others.

Lastly, I have had to accept that DM just isn't fair and it will never make sense. It just is. It appears that my last pregnancy triggered the DM for me. Different things seem to trigger it for different people. The trigger, if there is one, usually involves significant stress.

I would like to encourage any newly diagnosed person reading this to rise to the occasion and accept the challenge, no matter how hopeless or impossible it may sometimes seem. Because, one day, in the not-too-distant future, dawn will come. And with it, moments of clarity and joy. *Never stop coping. Life is worth it.*

I have faith in myself and in my humanity and in my creative ability to cope with life problems when they come. I do think it is perfectly normal that we will have mood swings and spells where we are very dark and gloomy and feel sorry for ourselves. Who wouldn't? We can be like the grapevine which twists and curls in all directions as it grows toward the sun.

—Donna Bueche, Illinois

DM Case # 16

Diagnosed Feb. 1998
Female

My journey started when I got sick in August 1996 after spending that summer trying to chase away a urinary tract infection. Boy, did my troubles ever get started!

I started with pins and needles in my hands, which progressed to zinger pains in my arms, feet, lots of fatigue, a very annoying cough, joint and muscle pain, brain fog. My ears would hurt for a few days for several months, but I forgot to mention this to the doctor as they weren't hurting when I was at his office.

My doctor ran tests and sent me to specialists. Nothing! This continued for a year and half, with symptoms coming and going. In February 1998 the doctor told me that even though the many tests didn't indicate it, I had a connective tissue disease. She began calling it RA, but it was really centering on it as a catch-all.

I went home and looked up RA on the Internet and found all kinds of things I didn't ever want to know. There was a web site - www.rheumatic.org" that was so different. It was brimming with Hope! Not a trace of "learn to live with the pain."

Since that was early in my diagnosis phase, I moved on. So far the tests hadn't indicated RA. That web site and their mention of something called Minocin stayed in my mind.

Back to February 1998, my doctor indicated that I had

a connective tissue disease. At that appointment, I was seeing her because I had an upper respiratory infection. She told me she wanted to treat the URI and the RA with an antibiotic called Minocin.

I rushed home to find that site on the web that had been so positive and full of hope. I thank God I found it.

The skeptical side of me kicked in. After all, this is the Internet! Can you believe everything you read here? Of course not!

The rheumatic web site looked good. The people appeared happy and trustworthy. But I still had doubt.

At that time there was a patient's conference led by Dr. Franco from Riverside, Ca. I signed up for it through the Internet. My skepticism was running on high gear. Finally, I thought, "If one of my kids was sick, would I leave any stone unturned in the search for an answer? Absolutely not!

At the conference were people from a support group. Dr. Franco fine tuned my diagnosis to DM. I came home full of hope and enthusiasm. I shared with my doctor all that I learned at the conference. I gave her a book, "The New Arthritis Breakthrough" by Harry Scammel!

After two months on the Minocin, I began improvement. My feet didn't hurt anymore! In September 1998, Zithromax was added to my repertoire. This helped greatly to control my cough, which was a major problem by that time. Little by little, there was improvement in my energy, pain levels, muscle strength. I am now at the point where I am back roughly 80-90% normal.

I went to an ENT doctor regarding my ears. The ENT said I might have another connective tissue disease called Relapsing Polychondritis. This set me back until some research I discovered indicated that Minocin can also be used for RP. The research was by Dr. David Trentham from Harvard University.

Here I am, getting better every day. My muscle strength has improved much. My college-age children reminded me that I had better rebuild my muscles if I wanted to be able to lift my yet to be conceived grandchildren some day. Talk about an incentive! I feel I have attacked this disease at it's source.

~

Thank you, Dermatomyositis friends, for taking the time to express your thoughts and experiences so that other DM diagnosed individuals may learn from you.

Chapter 2

POLYMYOSITIS

Polymyositis (PM) does not have the characteristic rash of Dermatomyositis (DM). Onset of muscle weakness usually progresses slower than DM. Proximal (nearest to the trunk of the body) limb and neck muscles are weakened, involvement of distal (farthest from the trunk of the body) muscle varies. Difficulty in swallowing is common in PM. Inability to breathe due to muscle failure is uncommon but occurs more often in PM than in Dermatomyositis or Inclusion Body Myositis. As many as one third of PM patients have muscle pain, but it is rarely a chief complaint.

Polymyositis literally translated means "inflammation of many muscles." Polymyositis (PM) is a disease characterized by generalized weakness - often without pain. The peak onset is between ages 30 and 60+. PM rarely affects people under the age of 20 but cases of childhood and infant Polymyositis have been reported. More women than men are affected with PM.

High dose Prednisone (an immunosuppressant) has been an effective treatment for many patients. Other immuno-suppressants such as Azathioprine and Methotrexate are used also. Unfortunately, these drugs have adverse side effects, especially with prolonged use. For patients who do not respond well to Prednisone, intravenous administration of immunoglobulins (IVIg) might be effective.

PM Case # 1

Diagnosed 1997
Female - Present Age 54

I was in the nursing profession for the greatest part of my life and at the age of 45 noticed that I just couldn't physically continue to do the work. I took some courses and got my real estate license and have had major financial success in that field, even though it was not my "first calling."

In 1973 at the age of 27 I was involved in a serious automobile accident (Myositis is usually brought on by some unusual trauma to the body) that caused me to be in a body cast and brace for about a year. After that accident, as I look back today, my body was just never the same. But at age 27, you never look back. You continue on that exciting trek to what will be your future.

I began to see muscle atrophy and have muscle weakness to a noticeable degree by the time I was 38, but my doctors assured me that it was due to my having been in a body cast and brace too long and that I needed to have surgery to remove some thickening on both sides of my hip/thigh area called a bilateral contracture tensor facia lata.

The surgery did seem to give some relief at the time, but I had begun having pain daily and taking pain medication along with steroids to "mask" the stiffness and to try to live a normal life, which was not to be. As I became weaker and less active, going to every doctor that I could to try and find out what this "intruder of life" could be.

In 1997 when I was making one of my routine trips to the emergency clinic because of a fall, the doctor that was on call suggested that I see a Rheumatologist. That was when I heard the word "Myositis" for the first time. Coming from a nursing background I recognized the word "poly" meaning "many" and Myositis meaning abnormality of the muscle. Little did I know what an innocent sounding diagnosis had done to my body over the past 20 years, but thank God, it finally had a name.

I had the first of two biopsies in 1998. The first one on the front of my right thigh didn't produce enough muscle fiber to be diagnosed. The second showed definite Polymyositis and I began taking Prednisone, which I now attribute with a great deal of memory loss, swelling and many more major side effects. My CPK was 2800 on one of my trips to the emergency room due to another fall. Because of the misdiagnosed CPK, I was taken to cardiac intensive care for a week.

The disease itself is hard enough to contend with, but the lack of knowledge about it and the lack of physicians who are adequately trained to diagnose it is the most frustrating part of Myositis.

I am beginning my second year of Methotrexate and still take the Prednisone, but I am down to an every other day dose. My energy is up some days and down the next. I know that I am supposed to be doing some kind of exercise but it is very hard to just do what is absolutely necessary to get from one place to the next.

It is the prayer of this group of people, bonded together by this horrible disease, that others will not have to suffer for as long as we have before being diagnosed.

Please join us in our efforts to let others know about the disease and encourage the medical community to spend more time and money in finding new and better treatment for the hundreds of sufferers of this
disease that are still out there wandering from doctor to doctor trying desperately to find out what is wrong with them.

Our prayers and our efforts are for you!

PM Case # 2

Diagnosed 1990-1992
Female-Present Age 56

While teaching young children I often found it difficult to get up off the floor. I was not sore and had no pain. I blamed my age and perhaps a few extra pounds.

A few minutes after school dismissed, we traveled by car to California. Repeatedly, it was difficult to get out of the car. Some days I would be fine. During the summer months I became weaker more frequently. Still not much pain.

I began with the family doctor. All X-rays of joints were fine. Blood tests showed everything within normal range except for the SED rate - over 80. My blood was sent all over the country for testing.. At that time doctors were sure I had Lyme disease, but the tests were negative. Next, I was sent to a physician who treats rheutoid arthritis. He thought the anti-inflammatory drugs would be the answer and that I would soon respond to one. However, not one of the medications helped my condition. He said on the next visit he would start *Gold Shots!*.

Luckily, I began to read and learn about gold shots. Nothing was wrong with my joints, so I would not return for that kind of therapy.

As I became weaker and the family doctor was ill, they referred me to a new young Internist. He gave me a dose pack of cortisone and the next day I hopped out of bed and baked cookies. But a few days later, my strength was gone again. So, he knew what would help me, but didn't know how to regulate it.

I was told to call Mayo Clinic and get an appointment. I would have arrived there December 23rd, but my family doctor mentioned about a physician on the edge of town who handled "weird cases."

When I staggered into his office, he said, "You have Polymyositis." I was so thrilled I cried! I had kept a diary of events and feelings. After talking with him, I had a muscle biopsy (right shoulder) which was sent to Baylor University in Texas. The test proved positive with the note that they thought I might be coming out of it and could possibly get well.

What this doctor prescribed was exactly like case studies sent to me from library resources. So I trusted his plan completely. He did not want me as a patient if I would not follow his plan. I was more than willing!

We began with Prednisone and Methotrexate shots. I do not remember the dosages but the strength of Prednisone was gradually reduced over two years. Time certainly helps with forgetting the days of inability to function

But many changes were to take place. First, I had to give up my teaching position. Then I thought I would read all the wonderful books I had collected. But I couldn't concentrate. Television wasn't an option as it made me very nervous.

As weeks passed by, I became weaker and weaker. My husband would dress me and get me on the sofa before he left for work. A few hours later I would roll myself to the floor and crawl into the kitchen where I could pull up to the island. I would rotate around it for a long time until I was limber enough to find something to eat. Then back to the sofa.

Some days were better than others. At times I was able to be in public and only close friends knew my real condition. Small muscle activity was easiest. I wrote letters constantly. We had a slide lock on the storm door and I had no strength to work it so I kept a hammer by the door to hit the slider to open the lock. Many days I could not open the car door, but if someone opened it for me, I could drive fine.

Pain began in my left leg, then moved to the right arm, then throughout the body. But it was tolerable. The weakness was much harder to tolerate. One day a friend came with a huge salad and I was not able to coordinate the utensils to get bite-size pieces. It looked like a huge obstacle to overcome. I was worn out before I began. The best way to describe me is to say I felt like I had been beaten and was trying to come out of a long period of suffering.

They told me to rest each day but it seemed more important to stay limber. Toward the end of my illness when I thought I was getting stronger I had a horrible spell of vertigo. It terrified me and I stayed home for weeks afterwards, never sleeping in bed, but upright in a chair with several pillows.

Slowly I came off the Prednisone and weekly shots. I was one of the lucky ones. My SED rate stays between 21 to 25. Daily I do water aerobics in 90 degree water. Doctors seem to think we will all end up with rheumatoid arthritis so I think staying limber is good. I can do most things. I cannot tolerate exercise equipment. Climbing stairs is very hard for me, especially if I am carrying a load. If I walk daily I pay dearly in the weeks ahead, feeling exhausted.

Prednisone was a wonderful drug for me. I didn't have highs or lows with it. I would take it again without hesitation. The weight gain is still with me, but I function once again.

Looking back, I believe that my problem started with a bad fall during the early summer weeks before my diagnosis. I know trauma to a body can cause odd things to occur. No one had addressed this, but I believe it can occur this way.

An older friend has Polymyalgia Rheumatica. An automatic train door knocked her backwards off a train and her back was broken. The pain and weakness of her Polymyalgia completely disappeared with her hard fall. I believe my condition was "set" off" by the trauma to my body.

I do not want this disease ever again! I aim to stay mobile, have annual blood work and pray for those with the disease. Some people do not recover. For special prayer about your condition, e-mail me at KakiOn@aol.com.

God knows your hurt and your heart. Give your load to Him and let peace be your focus. - Karen

PM Case # 3

Diagnosed 1977
Female - Present Age 54

Prior to January 1977 I had been feeling very tired and noticing some odd things with leg strength loss for several months and wondered why this was happening. Early in January 1977 I had progressed to being almost unable to hold a spoon to my mouth to eat and being fearful of driving my car as I couldn't lift my legs well. I could hardly turn over in bed and get out of bed.

After being diagnosed with Polymyositis, I was prescribed several medications including Prednisone, Imuran, Aleve, Verapamil (for Raynauds) and Didronel for osteo. These medications helped to some degree. The medication that *did nothing to help* was Methotrexate (up to 25 mg weekly).

At the present time, I use very simple medical aids for mobility and strength loss. If I choose to take a bath instead of the shower, I have to use grab bars installed in the tub area. As far as my strength loss since taking the medications and will probably never regain the strength in my arms, legs, back and neck. But, I am much better now than before being diagnosed and I function well in my "job" as domestic engineer with the exception of heavy housework.

I had to do some re-arranging in the kitchen cup-boards when I was able and always try to take things with me that belong in the basement when I have to go down there. I am fortunate that I don't really have to go into the basement if I don't feel well and strong enough to make the stairs.

Further, I made adaptations in things like lugging in grocery sacks when I was better, but still tire very easily on our four steps to get into the house by bringing the bags and sitting them on a planter around the steps. After putting the car into the garage, then slowly and carefully climbing the steps to retrieve the groceries bag after bag to get them into the kitchen. I conserve steps whenever, however I can because walking can be so strength-sapping.

But Polymyositis hasn't affected my tongue or the use of it!!

Since the beginning of my illness, long before I knew I was really sick, I never had the feeling of total devastation nor the "Why me?" question. I don't really know why, but perhaps because I've seen people and children with much worse things to face such as death.

I am working with a group since 1994 helping victims of the Chemobyl disaster and even prior to my diagnosis, I had adjusted any attitude I'd ever had about feeling bad about things.

We suffer not much in comparison to those poor folks. Plus, I have a very strong faith in God and have an extremely supportive husband and son. I am sure that has made all the difference in the world because I have their support, their under-standing and help whenever needed. Of course, I'm sure every one with a major disease will have family who have no knowledge of the disease and will not ever listen to an explanation, but there are family members who are very supportive, helpful, under-standing and caring.

One of my goals now is to help those with Myositis diseases and other diseases; encourage them as long as I am able. The Prednisone that makes me so puffy has bothered me the most and I have learned to "work around" forgetfulness somewhat, otherwise we all just laugh about it.

I am, of course, the perennial optimist and hope that my health won't worsen. I have always dealt with things as they happen and try not to borrow trouble before it happens. I would like to help educate people about rare diseases.

I have found great help with the various Internet web sites regarding the Myositis diseases and have met some wonderful people through that source. I actually have known for over 30 years someone with Dermatomyositis but each of us were told that the other had Lupus!!

Further, I also have true mixed connective tissue disease beside Polymyositis and I feel I've had that since 1988, if not before. My doctor agrees with me. In July 1998 my husband was diagnosed with diabetes insipidus, a disease even more rare that Polymyositis - even some medical professionals think it is diabetes mellitus.

So in the past few years I've learned more about medical stuff than I ever wanted to know. But, in my opinion, God has a plan in this and will direct both of us to be as helpful to others with these disorders as best we can.

It is astounding to me how many people I know among my friends and acquaintances that have some sort of autoimmune disease.

We could actually start a Prednisone support group almost in my church and among other close acquaintances!

PM Case #4

Diagnosed 1997
Female - Present Age 59

My name is Darlene. I am a 59 year old lady. When I was definitely diagnosed with Polymyositis in 1997, after a muscle biopsy, I was almost "happy." I had been seeing doctors for several years with terrible muscle and joint pain and weakness, and was just told that it goes with getting older. It was "just" arthritis and Fibromyalgia.

I was fortunate to have found a wonderful Neurologist, who is doing research into the Myositis diseases. She took great interest in my case. It finally had a name, and I could now concentrate on doing something about it (and, oh, how little that has seemed at times!) There are many days when it is difficult to get out of bed, but generally, it is a matter of difficulty climbing stairs, getting out of low chairs, walking any distance, or standing for any length of time.

I had already been taking Prednisone for "whatever" ailed me, and although the side effects were most unpleasant, the good effects outweighed the other. I knew I had to keep active and my answer and incentive was simple.

I had a dog who I loved with all my heart, and we were used to having two long walks every day. I was determined this would not stop, and no matter how much weakness and pain there was, I could not let "Zipper" down, and this was a promise I made to him and myself. I very rarely missed a day thereafter.

After having him for ten years, I lost Zipper to cancer last summer, and my heart was broken. But I tell myself he is still here needing me, and I very much still need him. So "Zipper" and I still go for our walks every day, although, I must admit, the challenge is much greater now ... with an invisible dog!

I eventually started IVIg (intravenous immunoglobulin) therapy, and I have been one of the fortunate ones. The physician provides me with six or so weeks of quality movement and decreased pain after each treatment. Even more so, psychologically these treatments have offered me a great deal of incentive, encouragement and inspiration in a strange way. I receive the treatments in a Medical Day Care Unit at a major hospital.

There are about two dozen patients in the unit at any given time for a variety of reasons. Many are receiving Chemo-therapy, marrow transplants, or other forms of help for potentially and likely terminal illnesses. A large number of these people are very young, but I have found they all appear to have one thing in common - *an incredible positive and cheerful attitude!* Although I do go through the "why me?" phase with Myositis, these brave people have made me realize how fortunate I truly am, and how little I have to complain about.

One of the most difficult aspects of the disease has been reaction of friends and family to the fact that I am no longer as active as I used to be, equating my inactivity to laziness. I don't like to rattle on and on about the problems with Myositis, and they are really interesting. But because I don't talk about it a lot, they don't realize how much pain I am in, or how difficulty it is some days just to get out of bed since the fatigue is so overwhelming. It is difficult for people to understand something they can't see.

My computer and the Internet have been blessings as they have allowed me to be in touch with other Myositis "victims" (my, how I hate that word), and we share encouraging words and thoughts. I don't personally know anyone else with the illness, so my "online" friends have been a blessing.

I daily try to maintain my sense of humor and a positive attitude. I do feel that with God's will, and the excellent medical attention I am receiving, the Myositis will be contained and not get worse. One of my biggest hopes is to be able to stop the Prednisone some day.

I have greatly changed my priorities. I no longer worry if the housework is not done everyday. I accept offers of help from friends and neighbors. I take long walks in the sunshine on the good days; shorter walks on the bad ones. I don't take to climb mountains, little hills make me just as happy.

PM Case # 5

Diagnosed 1997
Female - Present Age 49

I am a 49 year old female with Polymyositis. But, let me start from the beginning.

In 1994 I was living my life like a house on fire. I was the mother of two teen-agers. I was working full time at a large high school. Even though I had a stressful, high demand job, I loved it.

But I was just exhausted and struggling with feelings of depression. It was winter and my daughter and I had started going to the tanning beds. Big mistake! I developed a rash on my face that would not go away. I finally stopped by our little drop-by clinic, thinking I could pick up some ointment.

Being suspicious of the rash, they ran some blood tests and I was to call back for the results. I didn't. I didn't have time. Finally, they called me. I was 44 years old and diagnosed with Systemic Lupus Crythematosus.

For the next three years I struggled with fatigue, rashes, joint pain, and muscle pain. I tried working four days a week. I tried working three days a week. But try as I might, I struggled to keep going. The muscle pain continued. The high school where I worked was four stories high. It became impossible to use the stairs to get from one floor to the next.

In the Spring of 1997, I found a new doctor. He immediately ran a CPK test, ordered an EMG, and a muscle biopsy. My CPK was at 3600. I was diagnosed with Polymyositis and started on 80 mg of Prednisone. I thought, "Fine" and off to work I went.

Prednisone did a number on my head. I had difficulty organizing thoughts. I couldn't start at point A and get to point B. I wish I had been warned of these possible side effects. I might could have saved myself some humiliation.

In short, I was a mess. My doctor wrote a letter saying I was unable to continue in my current position.

I still have not returned to work (three years later). I have not found a way to deal with the fatigue, the muscle pain, and the lack of stamina caused by the Lupus and the Polymyositis. My CPKs have not returned to the high levels but are often elevated just above the normal range.

I take Prednisone off and on, depending on how my blood work looks. I have been on Plaquenil since 1994. I take Zoloft which has helped with the depression. I take Ambien to help me sleep. Daypro helps some with pain. So far, I have not found adequate relief from pain.

It has taken me a long time to acknowledge that I'm not able to handle the mental challenges that I once did. I get flustered and overwhelmed with the problem solving, organizing, conversation, study, etc. That has been a tough admission. We have agreed at my house not to discuss important issues late in the day or when I am especially fatigued.

One of the difficult things was finding a physician that I felt understood my illness and could explain it to me. I feel physicians tend to treat blood tests and I have found that the symptoms have a life all their own. There are days that it is difficult to walk or use my arms. Then, that seems to improve somewhat.

Then, there are days that I am absolutely overcome with fatigue; then days when it isn't so bad. There are days when burning muscle pain will put me to bed. Then, just when I think I can't take it, it seems to be better, only to return again.

This waxing and waning is terribly difficult. I don't think physicians take it seriously enough and relief from these symptoms can be hard to accomplish. Also, living in a world where we make plans and commitments becomes impossible. It is hard to be a dependable person and be totally undependable.

I have been fortunate in that I was able to accomplish many of my goals before I be- came ill. I was able to earn a Master's Degree and have a successful career. My children are now young adults and I am thankful that during their early years, I was disease free. We survived their teen-age years. My days are pretty much my own now.

I am just now reaching a place of acceptance (sort of). I have come to think that I will not be able to return to work.

I struggle to accomplish the day as it is. I believe that not pushing beyond my limits, getting enough rest, being able to stop during the day and sleep, if necessary, acknowledging the effects of medications (such as increased fatigue) are critical to my health. I believe that not working is just as important to my treatment as Prednisone.

Frustrations? Oh, yes! One of the big challenges is that my mind or my heart leads me to do something and my body refuses to follow. Then there is the feeling that questions what all those years of going to school and working what for?

Perhaps, I would have done things differently had I known where I would be today. Then, there is that nagging thought that says I may jeopardize our financial stability. Oh, and the ones that say, "Where will I be tomorrow?" "What does the future hold?" But, one of the hardest things of all, is just to keep going when I'm so tired and when I am in so much pain.

My hopes for the future? For myself, I pray that I can maintain the use of arms and legs, especially my arms. I hope to get pain under control. I want to love my life in spite of the changes in it because I know that I have been so richly blessed. I want to find contentment in the things I can do and let go of what I can't.

I hope there is a deeper understanding of these diseases, better treatment and the ultimate cure. I would like to see more research and am especially interested in twin studies, because I have an identical twin

All people should have the medical treatment they need. I am concerned when so many struggle to pay for medical care and even do without food. I would like to see a better process for disability claims. I think that often those with incurable diseases who are denied are on-going of medical problems. Often those who are denied are those that having the least amount of "fight" in them and need the disability funds most of all.

I have received tremendous support from my twin sister who said to me, "We will walk this road together." That statement carried me many days. I have also received support from those on the Internet who suffer from Myositis diseases.

And so, I say to the fellow sufferers, “We will walk this road together.”

PM Case # 6

Diagnosed 1996 - Male - Present Age 73

I am a male, current age of 73. My Polymyositis was discovered somewhat by accident as a result of an annual physical four years ago. At that physical, my blood lab work indicated a rather high LDH level. As a result of that reading, various additional tests were made.

For several months, the doctors were somewhat baffled as to the course of the problem. Ultimately, my CPK was checked and was found to be rather high (about 1400) and I was referred to a Rheumatologist.

I was told immediately that it was 50% certain that I had Polymyositis, a disease completely unknown to me. To confirm the diagnosis, I was to have a muscle biopsy, which, indeed, confirmed the diagnosis.

Looking back, I was beginning to feel that something was physically wrong with me. I had difficulty in getting up from a chair, rising from a kneeling position and walking up steep inclines. At first, I attributed this physical weakness to creeping “old age.” But just prior to discovery of the disease, I knew that my problem was more than just old age.

As to treatment, I was started on Prednisone, 60 mg/d for three weeks, then 40 mg/d for four months, then a gradual reduction to my current level of 6 mg/d.

After using the Prednisone for six months, then came a gradual reduction to my current level of 5 mg/d. The drug Methotrexate was added and I now take 20 mg of this medication once per week. During the past three years of treatment, my CPK levels have been reduced to about 180-280, which the doctor deems acceptable.

As to my physical condition, I feel very fortunate. I have had the disease for 3-4 years and am still able to walk without the aid of even a cane. I am not able to enjoy all of the physical activities that I did previously. But, at age 73, I can still walk in the malls, drive and enjoy a limited amount of gardening. I do feel there continues to be a gradual decrease in the muscle strength of my legs, but my arms are still relatively strong.

My disease did respond to a combination of Prednisone and Methotrexate. Unlike many others who have been treated with Prednisone, I did not suffer many effects from the medicine. The only side effect from the medication was a modest weight gain and a “moon” face, which disappeared as the dosage was reduced.

While Polymyositis can be very disabling to some, I was one of the fortunate ones who discovered the disease early and had good response to treatment.

Mcowdrey@airmail.net

PM Case #7

July 1997 - Female
Present Age 65

In the early part of May 1997, I developed stiffness in my legs. By mid June, the stiffness became a weakness in my muscles, climbing stairs was becoming difficult and falling down increased. In June 1997, I lost the ability to raise my arms above my chest level. I became a wheel chair patient; only two short months prior I was the image of good health.

In July 1997, I was diagnosed with Polymyositis. I had never heard of this disease until that day. Then began the “extensive” series of tests, looking for the trigger (i.e. cancer, etc.) I visited various doctors in Chicago, including Loyola University. These doctors confirmed Polymyositis through blood tests and muscle biopsies.

Treatment began at 40 mg/d Prednisone and Methotrexate injections weekly. My CPK numbers were dropping. In late November 1997, I fell, breaking my hip. I was in the hospital for three weeks. I learned valuable exercises and about a polished board (makes access easier getting from the wheel chair to bed, to chairs, etc.) while I was in the hospital. Why didn't someone tell me about the polished board before now? It is a God send. *(Editor's note: this is an oak board (called a Transfer Board) about 30" long by 8" wide, highly polished. It is available at all medical supply sources.)*

In early 1998, the Prednisone was reduced and I started on IVIG infusions at four weekly intervals for two days at a time. This treatment seemed to have no effect, except to leave me exhausted. On August 21, 1998, my husband and I sold our home in Illinois. We moved to Katy, Texas (near Houston), closer to our daughter and her family.

I started seeing several doctors in Texas (a Rheu-matologist and Neurologist). My treatment was changed. Methotrexate was discontinued and Prednisone was stepped up to 80 mg/d. Initially my CPK levels went down considerably, but not without the dreaded Prednisone side effects (i.e. puffiness, weight gain, moodiness, too many to mention).

I maintained the ability to raise my arms above the chest, but my big muscles are weaker. The Prednisone was then reduced to 80 mg every other day. Treatment with Azathioprine was added which resulted in my becoming physically ill. Treatment with Leukeran made me excessively tired (one day I slept the entire day away).

During 1999, I suffered more bad news, including two cases of the shingles and the forming of cataracts (Prednisone is the culprit) on both eyes. The shingles disappeared as quickly as they appeared, and the cataracts had been operated on.

I began an aggressive exercise program (including water walking) in 1999 as the Prednisone was reduced. Due to the erosion of the muscles continuing, we saw a low percentage of gain each week.

Unfortunately, the Prednisone was tapered too far down.

I suffered another flare in late 1999 (I had just gotten out of the wheel chair and was using the walker. Now, I was right back in the wheel chair.) The Prednisone and Cytoxan were increased. However, this particular flare-up was un-responsive to Prednisone and Cytoxan.

Plasmapheresis was started November 1999. This was over a five day period and this treatment showed a positive effect; my CPK levels began to fall again.

In December 1999, IVIg monthly treatments followed and are currently continuing. The current muscle recovery is about 2% per week. We are very careful not to taper the Prednisone level below the target zone of 20 mg/d. We are currently at 25 mg one day and 20 mg the next, along with a daily dose of 100 mg Cytoxan.

Polymyositis is an on-going battle! The evidence seems to point to the cause being a virus, hidden in the body, which becomes active in late Spring (my worse flares happen in May/June).

Here are the medications prescribed:

Discontinued/Tried -

Methotrexate (brand name Rheumatrex) Azathioprine Plasmatheresis (October 1999, used for five days only)

Currently Taking -

Prednisone (brand name Deltasone)
Cytoxan (generic name Cyclophosphamide)
IVIg (intravenous immunoglobulin)

A list of helpful aids for the battle —

Light weight wheel chair
Lift chair
Stable walker
Transfer board for movement between chair, bed, etc.
Ramps (installed on steps)
U Step walker
Extended grabber (reacher)

—Pat, Houston, Texas

PM Case # 8

Diagnosed 1987
Female- Present Age 60

Before getting to the details of living with Polymyositis (hereinafter referred to as "PM"), I should give you a brief background of myself. I'm a 60-year-old mother of two grown sons and I have a wonderful husband of 40 years. We've always had a wonderful life. For that, I give thanks every day.

When our youngest son was one-year old (1971), I developed Insulin Dependent Diabetes. I have no family history of this disease. I was a very thin person back then. It took several months for the diabetes to manifest itself to the point of hospitalization and starting on insulin.

You might ask, "Why are you telling me this? What does this have to do with PM?" I have only learned in recent years that insulin-dependent diabetes is also an auto-immune disease as is PM.

Fast forward to 1987. That winter I thought I had a bad case of the flu. When I finally went to the doctor, he immediately hospitalized me with "pneumonia." I was there 3 weeks, but a diagnosis was not made about PM until after I was sent home. Of course, at that time, like most people, I had never heard the word Poly-myositis.

My symptoms were fever, fatigue, congestion in my chest, pain all over my body. I could barely get up or down stairs, in or out of a chair. After going back to the hospital, I was given large doses of Prednisone.

I probably do not have to tell many PM patients what that means. Even though the steroids helped the symptoms, I am still struggling with the side effects of Prednisone and have never been able to get off this drug after 13 years.

I am presently down to 8 mg/d Prednisone, but have fought Adrenal Insufficiency many times, to the point of hospitalization four times. Because of the years of steroids, my adrenal gland cannot work on its own.

A couple of years after starting on the steroids, the disease flared again. This time I took extra-strength aspirin for the pain as most anti-inflammatories were not acceptable because of the side effects which I experienced. At the present time, I am taking Vioxx and it does help the pain and doesn't mess up my head or make me more lethargic than usual.

Also, as a result of the cortisone, I have Osteoporosis and have broken many bones. I'm holding my own in this department. However, last year was a very rough year. In January 1999, I had a seizure. This was a total shock; had never had this happen before.

My husband thought I was dead. Due to quick action on several people's effort, my next door neighbor, along with my husband, were able to get me breathing again until the rescue squad took me to the University of Virginia Hospital. I was then put on Phenobarbital and have remained seizure-free up to this point.

Within two weeks of this episode, I slipped and fractured my back. My shoulder was already fractured at the time of the seizure; so, as you can imagine, the first half of 1999 was very rough.

I have not addressed the issue that can be most worrisome - Pulmonary Fibrosis. Not all PM patients have lung involvement, but I do. So far, so good. While doctors who have never examined my lungs always get alarmed when they listen to my chest. Right now, my pulmonary doctor thinks I'm hanging in there. I don't have a noticeable problem with breathing. I just can't do a lot of things people my age are able to do.

I guess that is one of the hardest parts of this disease for me: Acceptance!

I must work hard at telling myself how well I am doing, especially when all of my friends are zipping around and doing most things that they've done all their lives.

I've had to learn to live with this "other person - the one who is 60 pounds heavier than the woman before steroids." I've had to learn to live with extreme fatigue that rest won't help. Pain, in some degree and varying places, never leaves my body. I never know when I'll have a bad day, or even why it occurs. One of my lines is “If I knew what made a good day, don’t you think I’ve had sense enough to do the same thing everyday?”

My husband took early retirement 5 years ago to help me and he has done a wonderful job. He is my real-live angel! I’ve had many prayers on my behalf and I know that helps. I do have a “Wonderful Life” and am grateful for each and everyday.

I don’t take things for granted and appreciate the sunrises, sunsets, the arrival of spring, the hummingbirds’ return from Costa Rico.

I have peace in my soul and I am glad to be alive!

PM Case # 9

Diagnosed Oct. 4, 1998
Female - Present Age 43

Hi, my name is Joanne Garrison. I am a 43 year old female with Polymyositis, which means “many muscles inflamed.”

If you’ve ever worked out and felt how heated, sore and achy your muscles felt; that is how I feel everyday. If you don’t have a Myositis disease, you will feel better in a few days. I won’t.

I can no longer do the things I enjoyed so much. I would love to be able to walk down a tree-lined street hand-in-hand with my husband, feeling the sun shining on my face, the gentle breeze blowing through my hair, or smelling the freshly mowed grass, and the fragrances of blossoming flower gardens. Taking a stroll on the boardwalk just before sunset, walking on the beach, feeling sand beneath my feet as the surf washes them; looking for sea glass and shells to add to my collection.

The pain associated with this disease is breathtaking most days. I do my best to ignore it. I must keep going, I must be strong!

I must fight this incurable disease with all my energy! I must do this not only for myself, but for my family as well. This disease does not only effect me, but all who are close to me and those who will come in contact with me daily.

I have a strong will to fight, survive and overcome the trials and tribulations of this disease, which comes not only from within, but from the people I love to surround me.

They stand by my side and encourage me to keep going when I feel like I can no longer do so.

But I am only human. There are some days when I shed tears, and I get mad at myself because I don't know if I am crying because I feel bad for myself or guilty about having to depend on people doing things for me that I have always been able to do.

I was always the type to do things on my own. I was quite independent. I have always prided myself on being a very strong person, physically as well as spiritually and emotionally.

But this disease can take a toll on you. I have a hard time doing and accomplishing the simplest things now. I think the hardest thing for me was to accept the fact there are certain things I can no longer do by myself.

There are things that I cannot change, but I can try to make something positive come out of something negatived.

I have always told my children, "Don't say I can't, always say I'll try!"

Since not being able to work anymore, I have had time to write my poems. In fact, I just had one published a short time ago. The book is called "Dawn of Inspiration." My poem (Family Tree) is on page 215.

But all in all, I have never lost my sense of humor. I love to laugh and make people laugh.

Remember this: It takes less muscles to smile than it does to frown, so I smile as much as possible.

PM Case # 10

Diagnosed May, 2000
Female

Although I am somewhat new to this whole kit and caboodle, I will share with you my story, so far.

I was diagnosed three weeks ago with Polymyositis. Until I was diagnosed, I had never even heard of this disease. I have been having problems for quite some time, but my family doctor never could find a reason for my strange ailments.

It all started with a weakening and aching in my fingers that eventually overtook my entire body. I was always tired to the point of dreading even getting up to go to work in the mornings as I knew I had an hour's effort in getting ready just to go to work.

I felt as if I needed a nap before even tackling the drive to work. My voice started leaving me for no apparent reason. I started experiencing coughing, choking and periods of not being able to catch my breath.

Of course, being a smoker also, I blamed these symptoms on that. After a while, I started to think that maybe I was crazy and felt as if my doctor was getting untrusting at my reoccurring visits.

It wasn't until the first of 2000 I decided to change doctors and, thank God, I did. After three rounds of blood work and an escalation CPK level every time (ranging from 500-1670 in three weeks), my new doctor sent me to a specialist.

The specialist ran more blood tests, and EMG, muscle strength tests and took X-rays. Finally, a diagnosis!!

I went last week for a muscle biopsy from my thigh and thankfully everything looked good with it. I am on 40 mg/d Prednisone right now and am starting to have less painful days.

The Prednisone also has it's downfalls as we all know. I suffer from sleepless nights, dizziness, nausea, nervousness, eyesight, memory and thinking problems, not to mention the constant craving for food and the lovely weight gain that has been sent my way!

I am constantly hot (living in Florida doesn't help, that's for sure!) And my family is considering wearing their winter clothes (in May) to combat my heat problems because of the air conditioning being so low.

I may have to relocate to the nearest nudist colony to get any relief!!

I rely on my strength to God and prayer to help me through every day and have a great support team with my family and friends.

Thank you for your interest in this strange disease, but thankfully, treatable disease. Having been diagnosed so recently, I will be looking forward to the publishing of this book.

- Melanie
Florida

PM Case # 11

Diagnosed Oct., 1998
Female - Present Age 53

In hopes of helping others who might find themselves in the same situation as I did, I would like to tell you a bit about myself. My name is Vicki, single, age 53 years young and live on five acres in Southern California. My family consists of my daughter, son-in-law and three granddaughters who live in Australia, as well as five Arabian horses and three mutt dogs.

I had never heard of Polymyositis until I was diagnosed with it in October, 1998. However, in 1995 I noticed weakness in my legs and trouble catching my breath.

I went to my primary doctor who ordered an X-ray and a sonogram of my heart. During that time, I was having a problem with my heart racing and skipping beats.

Later, this was diagnosed as a bad heart valve and I was put on a drug called Lopressor. Lopressor is used to lower blood pressure, but it also is used to regulate the heart valve. My normal blood pressure at the time was 85/60. Taking this drug lowered my blood pressure, making me very tired on top of my weakness.

As the years went by, my symptoms became worse and the weakness was more pronounced. In early 1997 my hands became painful. I was sent to rehabilitation for carpal tunnel syndrome treatment. I tried many times to ask questions and after awhile was immediately told that I was the patient and he was the doctor and HE would ask all the questions!

In December 1997, my symptoms had now begun very severe. I found it extremely difficult to breathe doing very simple tasks like getting dressed or brushing my teeth, but I passed this off as part of a flu bug going around. I started stumbling and falling although I had never considered myself old. I thought maybe old age might be catching up with me.

Finally, in May 1998, I made another appointment with my family practitioner. The doctor, after a blood test and X-ray, informed me that all my problems were due to a crushed disk in my neck.

As the days went by, I steadily weakened and it became much harder to breath.

My arms and shoulders became very painful to move. I had feelings of electrical shocks running down my arm muscles and at times I was unable to touch my own skin.

My hands ached and I had trouble using them. I had trouble sitting down and then getting up. I couldn't climb stairs and would have to stop and catch my breath after walking just 10 feet.

Vomiting was a daily event and every part of my body was swollen to twice it's size. My feet, legs and hands became huge. While I was eating very little, I continued to put on weight.

My doctor referred me to one surgeon who told me nothing was wrong with my neck. I went to another surgeon who said he wanted to put me in physical therapy for a period of two years then reevaluate me at the end of the period.

I went to Urgent Care twice. The first time I was informed since it had been an on-going problem that I needed to see my primary. I was getting sicker and weaker by the day now.

I tried to see my doctor again and was told I would have to wait another six weeks for an appointment. I returned to Urgent Care, It was on this visit I finally got some information. I saw a doctor who was very kind and after hours of waiting, he told me he suspected a Connective Tissue Disease.

I was told I have very little Potassium left in my system and I had abnormal protein counts, and had a lot of blood in my urine.

He wanted to admit me to the hospital but since it was up to my primary, he would have to call him. My primary apparently said NO. I had surmised this because the look on the doctor's face and the fact that the doctor said I had to see my primary the next day.

Before leaving Urgent Care that evening, the physician took me aside and told me to call 911 if I got chills in the middle of the night.

The next day the primary informed me that the Urgent Care doctor was way out in left field on his diagnoses and all I had was an allergy.

During my visits with these various doctors I was given a variety of reasons of what could be causing these symptoms (that it was all in my head), see if any of them sound familiar to you:

1. Maybe you're just going through the change.
2. You're just under a bit of stress.
3. Did you have a fight with your husband?
4. It could have been something you ate.
5. You must have picked up a little bug.
6. I think you just have an allergy.

After putting up with this for six months and hearing it was all in my head, I decided it was time to find someone who would listen to me and not patronize me. After asking for a transfer and without insurance for two weeks, I started seeing my new primary who is an Internal Medicine doctor at Scripps Clinic.

It didn't take Scripps very long to see that I was very sick and barely able to breath. After looking at the X-rays they had taken, an ambulance was called immediately, taking me to Green Hospital in La Jolla, Ca. This is where "Miss Poly" and I officially met.

I stayed in the hospital October 1-11, 1998. A muscle biopsy was performed to confirm what was already been suspected. To hear these words "You *have Polymyositis*" is overwhelming.

What is Polymyositis? Who else has this disease?

How did I get it?

Can it be cured?

How long will I live? Will I always have this pain?

A million and one questions ran through my mind. I did wonder how long I would have left and to what degree would the quality of my life be?

In November 1998 I had to return to the hospital for a lung biopsy and Interstial Lung was found.

I continue to do research on Polymyositis and all Myositis diseases in the hope of sharing this information with others.

Polymyositis, at the moment, can not be cured but it can be controlled. With new drugs coming out on the market, and the top rate doctors I have at Scripps Clinic, I expect to live a very long life.

In reading the Myositis Forum everyday, posing to it as well, there are individuals who are having similar problems as I once had but they have been unable find help.

This can be very frightening. It is a shame that our health care system has gone in this direction, giving the patients very little help or encouragement. This is not to say all health care providers are the same. But the number of uncaring, unsympathetic, irresponsible doctors is growing.

I ask you if you ask your doctor questions regarding your health? Get copies of your lab reports as soon as you can. Get a copy of your medical records every six months and make sure it's correct. If it isn't, take it back to the doctor and have it corrected.

This is our health we are talking about so take your health matters into your own hands.

After I ordered my health records from my last health provider, I was shocked what I found! False statements, medications I had never taken, the doctor stating I was recovering when, in fact, I was getting worse, falsely stating he recommended sending me to another doctor.

If you keep getting the run-around, GO TO SOMEONE ELSE! Keep looking until you find someone who will listen to you.

(By the way, I did not have a crushed disk in my neck nor did I have a bad heart valve. I had Polymyositis with lung involvement.)

I hope each one of you finds that one special, caring doctor who can put you on the right path.

PM Case # 12

Diagnosed 1998
Female - Present Age 48

I am a 48 year old single female, born and raised in the boroughs of New York City, who, in 1998, was diagnosed with Polymyositis.

I was moderately active all my life. Before this illness, I went to aerobics classes at least three times weekly. I had an excellent job and was employed by the same company for 29 years. My job was computer and data processing related.

I was a department manager for a large company in the securities industry (Stock Exchanges) and my work was extremely stressful, but I loved it.

Being a manager, I had to deal with numerous personalities along with daily production deadlines plus union and corporation problems. There were times I had to work 12 hours a day or more. Occasionally I was required to put in weekend work. The operation ran 24 hours a day and for 20 years I worked the 4:00 PM to midnight shift.

My job was very much my life. I never seemed to have much time to start a family. In 1998, that all changed!

The effects of the Polymyositis became so extreme physically and mentally that I could no longer work. In 1998 I went on Long Term Disability. In 1999, after 29 years of service, I was terminated.

******

The following is sort of a diary of what transpired before and after diagnosis. Some of the dates may be a bit off, but they are close enough.

In 1987 I came down with interstitial lung disease which was confirmed by a Bronchoscopy. At the time, I was told I was having an allergic reaction to my birds.

I remember not being able to lift my arms above my head and feeling like there were hands around my neck, choking me all the time.

I can't tell you if it affected my legs, but I could not take 3 steps without chocking from lack of oxygen. My oxygen level was down to 60%. It continued downward to 40% after the Bronchoscopy. Although it was an outpatient procedure, they wouldn't let me leave the hospital.

I don't remember if I was having swallowing problems, but I used to fall asleep sitting up and I'd wake myself with moaning sounds that I'd make in my sleep.

My mom was taking care of me at the time and she said she could hear the moaning in the middle of the night.

I ran a temperature from 99 to 102 degrees. I spent nine days in the hospital on IV Prednisone and with Prednisone, my lungs were back to normal.

I returned to work and my lungs have remained healthy. A doctor who specializes in Myositis disease has recently told me this was my first bout with PM.

I started noticing different symptoms in 1995. While caring for a very ill mother, I found at the hospital that it was getting harder to get up and out of chairs. I thought it was from sitting so much so I ignored it.

This was a very stressful time for me. My family left all important decisions to me, including putting my mother into a nursing home and whether to honor my mom's "Do Not Resuscitate" wishes when she was dying.

She eventually passed away peacefully. A month after she died, I was promoted and put on the midnight to 8:00 AM shift. I had a new crew who tested my authority and patience constantly and I had to fire a woman I had worked with 27 years because of her attendance problems. More stress!

Although I had worked nights for most of my career, I couldn't sleep during the daylight hours. These new hours were taking their toll on my body and health. I was exhausted but never complained to my superiors. I couldn't let them think I couldn't handle it.

Life went on. I got somewhat used to my new hours, but I began getting weaker. In 1996 I tried climbing up a 2-foot concrete wall and couldn't lift myself. I needed my brother to haul me up.

Boy, did I think I was getting more and more out of shape. I was always clumsy as a youngster and fell often.

As I matured, it seemed as if my clumsiness was subsiding. Then, in 1997, the falls began again. If I'd step on a pebble, my ankle would twist and I'd fall down so fast - not even enough time to put my hands out to catch myself. I actually smashed my face into the ground a few times, hurting my lip.

We'd make jokes about it, but for me, it wasn't funny as it was happening more often. I didn't feel right. I couldn't put a finger on what it was that was bothering me. In fact, I just didn't feel good.

I went to my physician of five years and without examining me, he told me I was getting fat and lazy, to go home and start exercising. I figured he's the doctor and he should know what he's talking about. So, again, I began to ignore my symptoms. I thought it was the crazy hours I was working and the lack of a good nit's sleep.

I started noticing when sitting at my desk, the muscles in my legs were constantly burning. I thought it was because I was sitting too much and I tried walking around the office more.

When I'd sit, I kept my feet raised. I developed what I thought was bad arthritis in my hands. They'd swell up and get so sore and painful that I could hardly bend my fingers or type. My left hand pinkie and ring fingers began feeling numb. I could not extend the ring finger on either hand to reach the top keys on my keyboard.

The problem got to a point where I could not get through a work day without taking three extra strength Tylenol every five hours.

Concentrating at work became harder. I was having problems completing assignments. The pain and burning in my muscles were constant and the falls were now getting worse.

The falls kept happening when I was walking my dog. I was getting frightened I would fall when a car was coming and not be able to get up in time.

Lifting myself up from the floor was getting impossible and my knees were becoming sore and scarred from the falls.

To this day I cannot kneel on my knees without excruciating pain. I'm not sure if it's from the PM or from the falls.

I went to Florida with some friends and we rented a minivan. I could not get into the back of the van. One of my friends would sit inside and pull me while another was in back pushing me.

It seems pretty comical at the moment and we laughed, but I think they were just as worried as I was. I started noticing it was getting harder to pull my legs inside my own car, a small SUV that is not high off the ground at all.

In January of 1998, I tried to run across a busy Manhattan street and couldn't. My legs refused to work.

I was finding it harder to get out of bed and out of chairs.

I could no longer lift my head off my pillows to rearrange them.

Sleeping was no longer a problem. In fact, I was sleeping too much.

PJ's caused so much friction on my blanket that turning in bed became impossible.

I didn't have the strength to pull up the blankets.

Getting in and out of the shower was scary.

Getting dressed was becoming more difficult.

I noticed when I swallowed, it would take two or three tries to get food down. I have always had a fear of choking and I chalked that symptom to that fear. I never realized it was part of the PM, not even after the doctors started asking me if I was having swallowing problems. I didn't realize it as a symptom until it subsided.

One day I was going down the steps of my apartment building when my legs gave out from under me. I sat right down on the steps. I got up, started back down and it happened again. When I got to the lobby, I stepped down another small step and went right down again.

There was a gentleman in the lobby getting his mail. When this happened, I imagined he must have thought I was drunk.

I realized something was seriously wrong and my whole body started to tremble. I didn't know what to do or how to approach my doctor with this information. My weakened physical state was becoming scary.

At my annual visit, I told my GYN about the problems I was experiencing and what my doctor had told me about being too fat.

Quite concerned, she referred me to a new physician. She was also concerned and did a complete physical along with blood work.

She also contacted a Neurologist and set an emergency appointment. After the preliminary physical examination, while I was still there, the Neurologist called my new physician and suggested that I might have an autoimmune disease.

It was the first time I had heard the word Poly-myositis. She arranged an EMG for the next week. I know this test is not pleasant but I was told it would not be painful at all.

Boy, what a lie! The electric shock portion of the test was a bit uncomfortable but not so bad. Then came the needles. When they were inserted into my skins, the pain was so intense I broke out into a cold sweat and became nauseous.

The needles in my thighs were also extremely painful. Needles in arms, hands, and back didn't hurt at all.

When the test was over and I was back in my car, I began to cry. I should never have gone for this test alone. I realize now that the intense pain was due to the fact I had PM very active at the time.

My second EMG a year later was uncomfortable but not painful at all.

The Neurologist told me the EMG strengthened her suspicions that I had Poly-myositis but a muscle biopsy would confirm everything.

I was apprehensive and did not want to do this. But in April, I had a biopsy of my right thigh. Although at the time of diagnosis, my CK was not very high (71). The symptoms, blood work, EMG and muscle biopsy all confirmed Polymyositis.

I was put on 60 mg/d of oral Prednisone. The doctors agreed that I should not be working. So, after three years on the midnight to 8:00 AM shift, I went out on a short-term disability.

Stress and physical exhaustion were something I didn't need in my life at this time.

After three months, there was a small improvement in my strength, but the muscle pain remained.

I began seeing a Physical Therapist who insisted I use a four-prong quad cane and sent me for "Range of Motion" therapy. I found the cane useful while walking, but was very uncomfortable on the handrails which I needed to prevent falls. It was easy to trip on the prongs of the cane.

When going down steps, I'd just throw the cane to the bottom of the steps so I wouldn't have to hold it while trying to descend steps.

In July of 1998, after minor improvement to strength and none to pain, I was referred to a Rheumatologist. My CK was over 800 now. I had a running temperature all the time between 99.6 and 100 degrees.

The Rheumatologist immediately put me on 15 mg of injected Methotrexate weekly with 2 mg/d of Folic Acid. About an hour after the first injection, I developed diarrhea. The Methotrexate was increased weekly until I was at 30 mg. The diarrhea intensified with the higher doses, lasting four or five days a week. Then heartburn set in. The diarrhea is so bad that sometimes the pressure I have to exert from getting out of a chair causes me to have accidents. My muscles are too weak to hold things. These accidents are happening way too often.

Medications the doctors have prescribed for this problem seem to have little effect. They had me increase my Folic Acid to 4 mg/d. Again, there was no affect on the diarrhea. My CP was going up and down.

The Rheumatologist added Araxa and I began vomiting. He stopped it and tried Imuran. Same problem with vomiting. I stopped the Imuran. I continue to take the Methotrexate.

My eyelids swell with fluid while I sleep. When I awake in the morning, I can hardly open them. They drain all day, long, tearing, irritated and bright red.

I experience numerous bladder infections at least once a month. I have also developed some incontinence problems. I'm not sure if it's the disease or the bladder infections. If I sweat, I develop fungus infections anywhere my skin touches skin (under breast, in groin, under arms).

I was rapidly gaining weight and developed Moon Face and a buffalo hump on my neck. I developed Acne (which I never had as a teenager).

My hair is falling out. I have insomnia at least three or four nights a week.

I experience cognitive problems (I can't remember how to get to the local store or doctors.) I'd get to my car and couldn't remember why I was there or where I was going. I am already at a loss for easy words, numbers confuse me. I totally lose track of time and now I am always late.

I am easily stressed and I panic under the slightest bit of pressure. Due to the side effects of the steroids, I have to take drugs for high blood pressure, diabetes, osteoporosis and heartburn.

All my doctors agree that I have to be removed from Prednisone. I'm experiencing too many side effects. The problem is every time we get below 20 mg, my CK rises and pain and weakness increase.

The Prednisone is the only drug that is keeping the PM under control.

In November 1998 my Neurologist started talking about IVIg treatments. After some discussions with my insurance company, we started them in January 1999.

Unfortunately, after six months of this treatment, except for a lot of problems with my veins, I felt no change in my strength or relief from my pain.

In fact, I experienced my worst flare ever right after receiving my sixth infusion (CK was up to 3744). The IVIg treatments were discontinued.

After 180 working days, short-term disability becomes long-term disability - if your company's LED insurance company agrees that you are eligible for it. I was. I also applied and was accepted after two attempts for Social Security Disability (SSD).

It is July 1999. Except for some minor improvements (falling incidents have decreased), I still felt pretty awful. I was now seeing a new Rheumatologist who changed the Methotrexate injections to 25 mg of Oral Methotrexate.

I am still having problems with diarrhea, but it has eased a bit. The heartburn has intensified. I got over the counter drugs of Prilosec for relief.

My CK, Aldolase and SED rates still haven't stabilized.

October 1999 the Rheumatologist started me on injections of Enbrel, 25 mg twice a week. I could see no difference in how I felt and my lab work did not improve. After six months, the Enbrel was stopped.

March 2000 I saw a Rheumatologist at the Hospital of Special Surgery in Manhattan who specialized in Myositis diseases. After examining the lab reports, he felt satisfied that my doctors were doing everything that he would have done. He did suggest an alternate steroid treatment that might lower my side effects - Pulse Therapy. I am now in the process of talking with my doctors and insurance company about setting this up.

It is now May 23, 2000 and I continue to do battle with this strange disease. I still don't feel well. I continue to show weakness in my legs, neck, back, hips and arms. The pain never goes away. Painkillers only take the edge off.

The low grade of fever continues, my CK, SED rate and

Aldolase continues to fluctuate. The falling incidents have eased up, but I think that is because I am being more careful when walking.

I have lost my job and my lifestyle has changed drastically. I thought I'd miss working, but I'm so uncomfortable from the pain and feel exhausted all the time. I know there is no way I could work.

Some days I wake up, have a bite of breakfast, take my medications, feel exhausted and return to bed to sleep for several hours. I often fall asleep in my chair during the day.

I used to enjoy going out with my friends, taking vacations, and traveled frequently. Now I am limited to my days shopping at the mall.

In the past, I would walk to larger malls and still have energy to spare. Now, I can no longer walk an entire mall unless I'm with friends and borrow a courtesy wheel chair from the customer services in the stores.

I do not have the strength to wheel myself so I always need someone with me when I use a chair.

Most days, the problem with diarrhea prevent me from straying too far from home. I still do my own food shopping, but I'm exhausted when I'm finished. Sometimes I don't believe I'll have the strength to get the packages into my car and the refrigerated things into the house. Later, I retrieve the rest of the groceries.

I still drive very short distances. I find it painful to keep my leg in one position on the gas and I'm afraid I'm not going to be able to press the brake hard enough to stop the car.

Because of my physical limitations, I have a woman to come in and clean the apartment. I can do some of the laundry if it isn't too heavy with linens and towels. I can not do the vacuuming, mopping or sweeping the floors. I can dust ok, but my arms hurt so badly when I have to hold them up.

I use paper plates so I don't have too many dishes to wash because standing at the sink hurts too badly

I have stopped wearing panty hose because it was exhausting, trying to put them on. I no longer takes baths because I can't lift myself up from the tub.

I had grab bars installed by the toilet, in the tub and

shower areas to help me lift or steady myself. Walking up steps is hard and exhausting. Walking down steps is frightening. I am always afraid I will fall and not have the strength to hold on to the handrail. If there are no hand rails, it is impossible to use the stairs.

The long walks I used to take with my dog are over. I just don't have the strength to go out and afraid of falling. Aside from some range of motion and stretching exercises, the dog walks and food shopping are my main sources of exercise now.

Some of my friends and family do not understand my illness and why I don't exercise more. They think plenty of exercise will cure me. They ask why I don't golf anymore, because, according to them, it is such an easy sport.

They do not understand why I cancel plans when I don't feel well. They don't understand I can't move fast and become impatient.

A close family member has told me that this is all in my mind. I believe from questions asked that others think I have lost it and don't visit them anymore. They haven't come to visit me. They tell me I live too far away. Does that sound funny to you? Not to me.

People can say the most hurtful things to me . I often worry that I might have done or made the same remarks to someone else that had an illness I did not understand. I try to be patient with family, friends and strangers, but it is not always easy.

I know there are many diseases to have that are worse than Polymyositis and I count my blessings every day that I am still here and can function as well as I can. Unfortunately, this disease is not well-known and doctors and the public need to be more educate about PM.

Sometimes I feel I have more knowledge about the effects of PM than my doctors.

Finding the bulletin board of the Myositis Association of America during the two years since the diagnosis have been helpful.

I'm not so frightened that I am alone anymore. I know that I'm not crazy when I tell the doctors about symptoms they say have nothing to do with PM.

I see other patients experiencing the same problems and symptoms. I only wish doctors would start reading those bulletin boards on the Internet what the patients are needing and asking for. The medical profession could learn much from us with a Myositis disease.

That is one reason this book should be so helpful to the Myositis patients and the medical profession.

Thank you for allowing me to tell my lengthy story. I hope it helps educate someone when they find they have Polymyositis and I hope it eases some of their fears.

PM Case # 13

Diagnosed 1997
Female - Present Age 33

Hello, there! My name is Suzanne Ranae Coulter. I was born June 4, 1967 so I will be 33 years old in 2000.

The diagnosis of Polymyositis was given to me in the fall of 1997, following three long years of dealing with a disease and, thus, symptoms that did not have a name.

My troubles first appeared after the birth of my daughter in July 1993. Following her delivery, I was tested for immunity to German measles as is common practice after childbirth.

When I was immune, I was given the vaccine. The only reason I mention this is because some research shows this as a trigger factor for getting a Myositis disease. In my case, I believe this to be true because my symptoms started soon afterwards.

The first symptom was recurrent urinary tract infections. They came back around every 30 days and because of this, I had to be on several different antibiotics. I also learned the comfort of cranberry juice which I still use today.

At this time I was a store manager at McDonald's which

meant I was scheduled 48 hours per week but usually worked 55-60 hours per week. Since I was in a high management position, it was difficult for me to take time off. I tend to neglect myself and I kept working while trying to fend off the urinary tract infections

In addition to this, I had a family, a husband, a three year old son, and a newborn daughter.

Eventually, something had to give and it ended up being my body. I grew more and more physically tired. Then, one night, as I laid down in my bed, I realized I could not feel or move my legs. Terror swept over me!

That night in June 1994 was the beginning of something very frightening and life altering. I was admitted to the hospital but none of the doctors could tell me what was happening. They also could not tell me if I would ever walk again.

A Neurologist was called in to see if he could find out what was going on. He ordered lots of tests, including a MRI of my spine and brain and a spinal tap. He couldn't find anything wrong. So he started to treat the symptoms without a cause.

His course of treatment was high does of intravenous steroids (Prednisone) and when I could move my legs a little, then physical therapy. He wanted to send me to a rehabilitation center where I could get one-on-one therapy, but I had a different agenda.

I needed to be home for my daughter's birthday. So I walked the hallways of the hospital and progressed enough on my own until I was released to go home.

My strength was not normal, but I was home! I stayed home until after my daughter's first birthday. But because the steroids were tampered off (decreased) too quickly, I ended up in the hospital again in July 1994.

I could not walk again and I was also very weak in my arms and neck area. Of course, treatment was the same as the previous time except the steroid tapering was done more slowly this time.

The Prednisone has brought back my ability to walk and function, but it had also brought a lot of side effects. I gained 60 pounds and I looked like a "puff ball" with a round moon face. I was relieved to be tapering the Prednisone down.

I returned to my job as Store Manager in October 1994 after months of being off work. I had to take it easy which meant altering my activities both at work and at home.

Asking for help from my family and co-workers became a necessity and this was enough to sustain my physical strength for awhile.

Mental strength was another matter. I was worried about my future and my family's future. I had no answers as to why I was being paralyzed and I was not satisfied with that. I changed Neurologists in hopes of getting a second opinion and a name for these symptoms.

I research all the medical looks in the libraries and around the Cincinnati area. The closest diagnosis I would find was Lyme disease or possibly Multiple Sclerosis.

My new doctor ruled out Lyme disease because the tests were negative and MS was ruled out because the EMG showed muscle deterioration, not nerve damage.

The Neurologist was persistent and aggressive and ordered several blood tests and eventually a muscle biopsy which finally gave a name for my symptoms: POLYMYOSITIS.

In the midst of all the testing, I had changed jobs from McDonald's to Wendy's in hopes the change would help me physically.

But, fast-food is tough. No matter which restaurant it is. Wendy's did enable me and my family to buy our first home, but with the stress of the new home and the stress on the job, my physical strength was diminished and once again I was back in the hospital.

This time it was worse. Not only could I not move my legs, I could not move my arms, and my breathing was very labored and difficult. The steroids helped me again. I finally decided it was time to get away from fast-food. I tried retail management instead.

With a name for my symptoms, I set out to find any and all information about Polymyositis. I could not find much. I wrote MDA and various other associations and read all I could find in the libraries. Because of the versatility of the symptoms with each individual patient, it was difficult to plot the correct treatment for me.

My doctor suggested switching treatments. The steroids were not helping me enough to justify the side effects of the medicine. He thought we should try IVIg (Intravenous immunoglobulin).

For me, the IVIg is a five day treatment and, even though I take preventive medicine, I usually get an awful headache which leads to vomiting and diarrhea can only be stopped by taking Phenergan suppositories.

As a result, I get incoherent for a few days. Thus far I have been able to get the IVIg treatments in my home, however that could change with the new insurance company.

Since I am not bedridden, they may require me to go to a hospital as an outpatient basis, or they will not pay for it.

We do not have an extra $10,000 laying around to pay for the treatments on my own.

When I began the IVIg, I had to get a treatment every 4-6 months. This was when I was working at the retail management job. Since that job, I have taken a job as a 911 dispatcher. There is lots of mental stress on the job but no physical stress. I sit for a living now. Because of this, I have gone almost one year without the IVIg or any other kind of treatment.

I have learned to watch my physical stresses and I have learned my limitations. If I feel tired, I rest. If I feel back pain or weakness (which is how my relapses begin) I rest. If I do a lot of walking, I rest. I have altered my physical lifestyle and have no need for mobility aids or medicinal aids.

I feel a little unsure about the future at times, but I am also hopeful because I am walking. I look normal even though I have this terrible disease. That helps me to press on with my daily life.

In those times when I feel like giving up the fight, my husband is there encouraging me. I know my family loves and needs me, just as I love and need them.

I am fighting and adjusting and altering my symptoms so I can have a long joy-filled life. In the event I have another exacerbation, we, as a family, will once again fight and adjust and alter.

- Suzanne R. Coulter
304 S. Ash Street
Bethel, Ohio 45106
E-Mail: shecat67@aol.com

PM Case # 14

Diagnosed April, 1996
Female, Present Age 48

My symptoms started in September 1995. Coincidently, the same time that I took up golf and six weeks after sinus surgery. My goal in golf was to hit the ball forward; I didn't care how far.

This was the advantage of being a novice. I didn't have anything to compare it to and I needed to keep my body moving even if it hurt. I couldn't make a fist, but I could hold the golf club. I usually play nine holes walking and pulling my cart.

The Rheumatologist who diagnosed my disease is a golfer. We had a ritual that before he would look in my file for my current CPK, he would ask me how far I was driving the ball. My reply would usually track with my numbers: if I was hitting good, that would be reflected in a decrease in my numbers. If not so good, my numbers would be elevated.

Getting dressed was my most challenging activity. I would become so tired I would have to rest two or three times from showering to completion. Putting on panty hose was impossible so I switched to long skirts and knee highs. Many days I would forgo blow drying my hair and opt for the natural look. My husband would hook my bra for me and help with buttoning.

I am a lobbyist in the State Legislature and move to the capitol city during the session. Upon returning home from the thirty day Legislative session, my husband was hooking my bra and suddenly asked, "*Who has been doing this while you were gone?*" I then had to explain that it could be hooked in the front and twirled around in the back, although it doesn't twirl very easily!

That first Legislative session after I got Polymyositis was very rough. I was afraid I might not be able to stand up to the rigors of long hours. I also had gotten carpal tunnel syndrome and difficulty holding and carrying my files around all day. I thought I might have to get a helper dog with saddle bags to carry my things.

I had to quit taking the stairs. It not only took too much energy, I slowed everyone else down by taking a step at a time, bring both feet together before I proceeded to the next step.

By 1997 I also had bouts of shortness of breath so I just stayed off the stairs at work. I do live in a two story house and get exercise there.

Prior to being diagnosed I started going to acupuncture to help with pain relief. I was already going to massage therapy. I continue going twice a month to acupuncture and massage therapy.

When my doctor prescribed Prednisone, he told me about the weight gain, facial hair, and the other potential complications. I went to electrolysis for the facial hair, started calcium and multi-vitamins, got bone scans and counted my lucky stars that I had a loving husband.

In 1997 I went through menopause. A friend sent me a book about the different hormones and the kind of hormone supplements avail-able. They mentioned in one sentence that DHEA was being used experientially to treat Lupus disease.

My OB-GYN at the time (I have since changed) was uncooperative in working with my female and Polymyositis problems. My golf playing Rheumatologist said it was okay to take DHEA as long as I got it monitored in my blood tests. The blood tests reported my DHEA was low and I started by taking 150 mgs (normal dosage is 25-50 mgs) with a blood test. six weeks later. I remained on DHEA for two years, tapering off with blood tests every six months.

My CPK numbers did not go down during this period, but I don't know whether it was the DHEA because I also started taking Methotrexate at the same time.

Now, four years after my diagnosis, I have tapered down to 2.5 mgs every other day of Prednisone and 6 tablets of Methotrexate a week.

I have lost 32 pounds that I had gained. I rest when I am tired and I am very active in my community and travel as much as I can afford.

I do not want to say someday that I wished I had done something while I was still able to do it.

PM Case # 15

Diagnosed 1993
Female - Present Age 65

I am a 65 year old female who was diagnosed with Polymyositis at age 58. Before discovering the Polymyositis, I was originally diagnosed with Rheumatoid Arthritis and Sjogren's Syndrome at age 54.

After years of trying different prescription medications, mostly Prednisone, physical therapy and leg exercises, the Rheumatologist sent me to a Neurologist. He was able to confirm through nerve and muscle testing and a thigh biopsy that I had Polymyositis.

His assumption was that Polymyositis is occurring as a complication of the Sjogren's Syndrome. After this diagnosis was made, my Rheumatologist suggested a treatment of intravenous immunoglobulin (IVIg), but insurance companies rejected the treatment.

As for my physical limitations, my arthritis is in remission now. The problems I have with the Sjogren's Syndrome have remained the same over the years - very dry eyes (no tears), very dry mouth which causes tooth decay and cavities

(no matter how well I brush and take care of my teeth.)

I have participated in several studies at Southwestern Medical Center in Dallas and tried several artificial salivas, I discovered that using lots of artificial tears for the dry eyes and drinking lots of water and eating sugar-free hard candies for the dry mouth are helpful to me.

My physical limitations related to Polymyositis increased gradually for several years, but are not getting any worse at this time.

Two years after diagnosis, I began having difficulty in swallowing for several years. I had my esophagus dilated (stretched).

The first attempt could not be completed because they did not have a tube small enough to use. I returned later to the hospital for this treatment when an infant tube was located. After the procedure, I have had no more problems with swallowing even though the doctor said it might have to be done again in the future.

I have difficulty rising from a sitting position, especially from a soft cushion. I have found that wearing only low heeled shoes helps in getting up. It's also very difficult to rise from a toilet.

Some of my worse experiences have been in rest rooms that aren't equipped for the handicapped. I was once stuck in a stall for 15 minutes in A MEDICAL FACILITY of all places! I was in the lab for blood work and a urinalysis.

If you ever get stuck in a stall without bars, you push yourself up with one hand on the wall behind and the other hand on the seat, if necessary. At home I recently installed a taller handicap style commode that is much easier to rise from. I can't squat down to the floor. If I somehow wind up on the floor, I have to crawl to a piece of furniture to hold onto and pull myself up to my feet.

For the first three years after diagnosis, I would only take showers, not baths, because I couldn't get out of the bath tub. I learned how to take a bath again by getting on my knees, pulling myself out of the tub by pushing against the wall and holding onto the shower door.

I also occasionally drop things when I thought I had a

firm grip on them.

Although at times the frustration of coping with this disease on a daily basis is over-whelming. I have been determined to find ways to overcome the problems I face with the help of my greatest support team - my family.

Thank you, Polymyositis friends, for taking the time to express your thoughts and experiences so that other PM diagnosed individuals may learn from you.

Chapter 3

Inclusion Body Myositis

Inclusion Body Myositis (IBM) is very similar to Polymyositis. In fact, many doctors believe patients diagnosed with PM that do not respond to treatment actually may have IBM. The only definitive test for IBM is a muscle biopsy.

Onset of muscle weakness in IBM is usually very gradual, taking place over months or years. It is different from PM in that both proximal and distal muscles are affected. Typical findings include weakness of the wrist flexors and finger flexors. Atrophy, or shrinking, of the forearms is characteristic. In the legs, Atrophy of the quadriceps muscle is common in varying degrees of weakness in other muscles. Difficult swallowing (Dysphagia) occurs in about half the patients with IBM. Facial muscle weakness is present in a minority of patients. Many times falling is the first noticeable symptom of IBM. Some patients have no pain; others have tremendous amount of pain.

Fine motor movements such as lifting any flat item - pencil, paper, etc - from a desk or floor, buttoning a shirt, zipping pants, sewing, writing and even the ability to take care of personal hygiene or feed themselves as the disease progresses, encompassing the necessity of help in dressing, tying shoes, even showering. A use of a wheel chair or scooter for mobility becomes absolutely necessary after the canes and walkers aren't useful anymore.

Symptoms of IBM usually begin after age 50, although no age group has been entirely excluded. IBM occurs more frequently in men than women. About one in ten cases of IBM may be hereditary.

Unfortunately, there is no known treatment for individuals with IBM. Intravenous immunoglobulin (IVIg) has shown small improvement to patients in the treatment of IBM.

Strength allowing, prescribed physical therapy may be helpful to maintain mobility.

As this manuscript was being written, Dr. Richard Barohn, Chief of Neurology at the University of Texas Southwestern Medical Center, sent a note to me. He and Dr. Anthony A. Amato have completed an IBM study February 3-17, 2000 for "The Current Treatment Options in Neurology."

This is the Opinion Statement of the Study:

> "Inclusion Body Myositis (IBM) is usually refractory to immunosuppressive therapy: however, a few reports suggest that a minority of patients with IBM may have a partial, transient response or that therapy may slow progression. Therefore, although we generally discourage the use of immunosuppressive therapy for IBM, if the patient is willing to accept the potential side effects of therapy, a 3-to-6 month trial of oral Prednisone can be attempted: 100 mg/d for 2-to-4 weeks, then 100 mg every other day for 2-to-3 months
>
> "If Prednisone alone produces no improvement after 3 months, oral Methotrexate can be added: 10-15 mg/wk for 6-to-12 months. If there is no objective clinical improvement in strength after a trial of Prednisone alone or Prednisone plus Methotrexate over the course of 6-to-12 months, we discontinue pharmacologic therapy. Because of the great expense, relative lack of availability, and minimal evidence of intravenous immunoglobulin (IVIg), we do not recommend this form of immuno-modulating therapy for IBM."

(Editors Note: We are grateful and fortunately to have Dr. Richard Barohn and Dr. Sharon Nations from the UTSWMC and Dr. Alan Martin, Texas Neurology, involved in our Myositis Support Group in Dallas, Texas.)

In addition, it is our pleasure to have the encouragement and participation of Dr. Aziz Shaibani, Director of Nerve & Muscle Center of Texas, Houston, in the development of this book about the differences among the Myositis patients, the differences about the treatments, and the differences among the medical professionals about the mysteries of Myositis. He submitted the following concerning IBM and IVIg treatment.

> " The story of Inclusion Body Myositis (IBM) is still evolving and the role of IVIg in it's treatment is controversial. I have patients who are doing well on this treatment. Study conducted in the National Institute of Health (NIH) revealed some encouraging results and need to be reproduced. The issue is that most patients with IBM are diagnosed LATE. With increasing awareness and the availability of neuromuscular centers, I hope this will change. Most of my IBM patients who responded to IVIg treatment were diagnosed EARLY. As you know, EARLY in the course, there is inflammation, while LATE, degeneration predominate the picture. During the inflammatory stage, treatment may be effective."

- Dr. Aziz Shanibani
Director of Nerve & Muscle Center of Texas, Houston

IBM Case #1

Diagnosed - 1992
Male - Present Age 59

"I used to think IBM was just a computer company."

December 19, 1992, my wife and were elated... I didn't have ALS. We had a party inviting all of our friends, after all, how bad could this IBM disease be?

My journey began in August of that year when being examined by a doctor friend concerning some cracked ribs. Casually, I mentioned that for some time I had not be able to make a fist with my left land. After an EMG my friend said I had something seriously wrong, giving me the worst case of dry mouth in my life. The diagnosis wasn't known but ALS was mentioned. My Rheumatologist (the next doctor in line) ruled out PM but also mentioned ALS,

The Neurologist also didn't have a diagnosis, mentioned ALS and sent me to the University Hospital. Four months later I see my Neurologist, he mentioned ALS, prescribes another EMG followed by a muscle biopsy. The results were noted and I was diagnosed with IBM, a non- threatening muscle disease with no treatment. My doctor wouldn't prescribe Prednisone because "it wouldn't help." I had turned 52 the previous month.

D+1 (First year after diagnosis): Life went on pretty much as normal, working, same hobbies and learning IBM could be an inconvenience at times. Read "*When Bad Things Happen to Good People.*" - excellent book. Started taking DHEA, vitamins and eating more green vegetables. Bought a "Lifecycle" and began peddling 30 minutes every other day along with lifting weights. Slight problem: getting up from chairs. Discovered IBMA that fall and called Betty Curry.

D+2: Bought a "neat" cane. Chairs without arms are out of the question. We fly to Hawaii for a great vacation. Unable to walk on the sand without help or get up from beach chairs - would've loved to swim in the ocean "for old times sake" but didn't think I could handle the low surf. Really tough climb up the ramp into our jet - learning to hate stairs. Heard about Coenzyme Q10 and L-Carnitine and start taking large doses. Selected for a research protocol at the National Institutes of Health in Bethesda, Maryland. I'm excited! Another biopsy con-firms my diagnosis and I learn I've had this disease since at least 1983. Also being a "left sided" disease - my left side is much weaker than my right side which includes my mouth and tongue.

During my four trips in five months to NIH, I was put on 60 mg of Prednisone a day and four "massive" infusions of IVIg. Met my first fellow IBM patient; I was no longer alone! NIH was overall, a wonderful experience.

Added bars behind and on the wall next to my toilet

Started wearing lighter shoes, Rockports and finally Ecco's.

Feet started swelling - support stockings really helped.

Visited a hardware store looking for anything that could help in daily living; found some 2" rubber coated hooks which were great for opening doors and drawers.

D+3: Bought a stair lift for our home - opened up our lower level once again and my computer. Was using cotton gloves with a rubber palm to help me hold on to the banister - worked for a few months.

Also bought a lightweight wheelchair just in case I would need it. Talked with a guy in a wheelchair who had been in a motorcycle accident 15 years before and from that moment, a paraplegic. I'm very fortunate as I've been given the change to get "used" to disability at my own pace.

We take a cruise to Mexico. Went very well. Attend MAA conference in Orlando and rent a scooter (even though I didn't need one) - loved the freedom it offered and ordered one upon our return home. My fingers were getting very smooth.

D+4: Visit with a guy with MS and try his light weight arm crutches - really stable! Have an appointment with a DO (Osteopath) for a try at "alternative" medicine. He prescribes injections of vitamin "K" and testosterone for a month - as with everything else I had tried to date. No help!

Getting in and out of the shower is getting difficult. Buy some light weight arm crutches just in case! Trade my favorite pickup truck for an SUV (Jimmy). Easier to get in. Have a lift installed to transport my scooter - if I need it! Had a link removed from my watch band.

D+5: Son-in-law builds a ramp so I can take my scooter outside - great timing as I could no longer climb the two steps from the garage. I had installed two drawer handles on either side of the door jamb and that worked for two years. Took a bad fall upon leaving a dinner reaching for my cane. Time for the crutches.

Sold my business and we move into a single level home already ramped and with a roll-in shower - HUGE change for us! Now I can use my scooter inside. Get "chilled" very easily.

D+6: Take a wonderful trip to England. Not very accessible, but enjoyed every moment. Walking less and less. Love my scooter and buy a used one out of our newspaper for outside use.

Spend lots of time at my computer, reading and watching sports on TV. Still go into work 2-3 days. I've been on SSD for a year and now I'm on Medicare.

D+7: Cruise to Alaska with 16 friends, rent a scooter for the ship. Worked out well. My shower's are very fast (too fast). Purchase a shower seat which solves the problem when grab bars are installed to the walls.

Visited Dr. King Engel (IBM expert) in Los Angeles. He wants me to try low dose Prednisone (20 mg every other day) along with the L-Caritine and Coenzyme Q10 for three months. No changes noted!

Getting very difficult turning over in bed at night as well as combing my hair (but that's a problem that's taking care of itself!). Haven't been able to dress myself for over a year. Of mankind's inventions, my least favorites are: steps, chairs, low toilets, zippers, buttons, shoe laces, pant's pockets, dull knives (I've carried an extra sharp pocket knife when we're dining out for many years) low car seats, pens (unless they are flat), spray bottles (I use "travel size" for everything) - a never ending list!

Recently, we purchased a new mini van and had it "converted," making traveling much easier. Also Medicare bought me a "Jazzy" power chair which is fantastic. I can still drive; for now.

I'm on no medication except for high blood pressure, a side effect from the first Prednisone usage. I have no illusions concerning my future!

My journey through this disease would have been difficult (early) and now impossible without the love and unselfish support of my wife. Also having the financial resources for which I am truly thankful. I strongly believe that getting the necessary equipment and assertive devices *before* you need them is a huge benefit because it gives you the option of "looking around."

IBM, like everything else in life, is indeed only a "temporary" condition and should not receive any more "special consideration" than those positive events that have added to our lives.

- Brad Bent - Colorado Springs, CO.

IBM Case # 2

Diagnosed 1998 - Male Present Age 45

I received a definite diagnosis of Inclusion Body Myositis in March, 1998 at the National Institutes of Health in Bethesda, Maryland. I am a 45 year old male and have been having symptoms of the disease since approximately 1991.

The diagnosis came after several years of uncertainty and mis-diagnoses. The first symptom I noticed was weakness in the quadriceps around the age of 36. I had noticed problems trying to jump, paying basketball or volleyball, and later, as I was coaching my son's baseball team, my knee would buckle as I was running bases.

For a while I put this off as being out of shape, but the weakness progressed to point I was having trouble climbing stairs and getting out of chairs by pushing with my arms (this was not long after I built a two story house with all the bedrooms upstairs!).

In the fall of 1994 I went to my family doctor for a physical, and explained the problems I was having with my legs. He examined me, had me try to rise from a chair and squat down in the floor, and told me I was now 40 years old and probably just out of shape. He told me at that time he knew of no diseases that just affected the quadriceps, and I was showing no weakness in other areas.

My wife is a nurse. When I discussed with her the doctor's conclusion, she encouraged me to get a referral to a Neurologist. I first went to a Neurologist in the city where I live. He ordered an MRI, and when that showed no problems with my spine. He conducted an EMG and nerve conductive study. He then suspected what he called an "Anterior Horn Cell" disease. He referred me to a Neurologist at the University of Virginia Medical Center.

In February 1995 I had my first visit with two Neurologists at UVA. They conducted a full EMG and nerve conduction study, along with a clinical exam that took most of that day. At the end of the day I was told that they had noticed some weakness in the upper body as well as the problems I had described with my legs, and they suspected a neuro-muscular disease.

They thought at the time that I had Spinal Muscular Atrophy or possibly Amyotrophic Lateral Sclerosis (ALS or Lou Gehrig's disease).

They told me there was no medication available for either disease, but put me on high doses of Vitamins C, E. and Beta Carotene. I had several other office visits with these Neurologists, and in July of 1995 I was told that they were changing my diagnosis to ALS.

This was a very difficult time that was made easier by the prayers and support of my family and friends. I was very encouraged by the phone calls, cards and letters I received during this time.

During the two years that I carried the ALS diagnosis, I applied for and was accepted in a "compassion program" through the National Organi-zation of Rare Diseases that allowed me to take a trial drug for ALS. This offered some hope, but made no change in the progression of the disease.

In June 1997, the Neurologist that I was seeing at UVA told me that because of the way the disease was progressing, he suspected that I did not have ALS, but possibly Inclusion Body Myositis. He asked if I would agree to another EMG and nerve conduction study. I agreed. After performing them, he told me that I should have a muscle biopsy and try to get a definite diagnosis.

A biopsy of the left deltoid muscle was done and two weeks later the doctor called me at home and told me that while the biopsy was inconclusive, he was still suspecting that I had IBM. He basically explained what IBM is and how it progresses, and gave me the name and address of the Myositis Association of America and suggested that I contact them for their literature.

By this time I had progressed to the point that I could not run at all, could not climb stairs without handrails, and was falling much more often. I also had a lot of trouble getting up after a fall. In the fall of 1997, my doctor arranged for me to be seen at the National Institutes of Health. My first visit was in February of 1998. Two Neurologists, who again ordered an EMG, nerve conduction study, EKG and blood work, examined me. They also performed a clinical exam. After viewing the results of the tests, they asked me to come back for another appointment, and another muscle biopsy, this time of the biceps.

Several weeks after the second appointment, I received a call at work from one of the NIH doctors. He told me the biopsy was conclusive for Inclusion Body Myositis. While I still did not know a lot about the disease, that night my wife and I had a celebration because we then knew it was not ALS.

For the two years since my diagnosis I have continued to be seen by the Neurologists at UVA. I continue to take the vitamins, and have added L Carnitine and Coenzyme Q10. My doctor gave me the option of trying Prednisone, but did not encourage it because of the very limited success with IBM and the side effects it has.

He called in an Endocrinologist and we started a regimen of testosterone injections to try and strengthen the healthy muscles.

While this has had no effect on the diseased muscles, I think it has helped strengthen the healthy ones.

I am able to continue working full time due to having a job where I can stay at my desk for most of the day. I am walking with the aid of a cane, and have to continually guard against falling.

The weakness has spread to my arms, fingers, and just recently started to affect my throat such that I have some problems swallowing. After facing the possibility of having ALS, I am very thankful for the gift of LIFE! My friends and family have been very supportive.

My employer has been very willing to work with me in any way they can. My wife, who assists me with many things, has been a constant source of strength and support through this ordeal. I am still able to attend and be a part of the many activities that my two children are involved in.

I have attended two of the MAA conferences, and have met some wonderful people, several of which have become good friends. I don't know what the future holds, but I continue to trust God to give me strength to get through each day. My hope and prayer is some day we will see a cure for all of the Myositis diseases.

- Gary, Virginia

IBM Case # 3

Male - Present Age 63

A Myositis Patient's Story from the United Kingdom

My name is Bill and, with a few exceptions that I won't mention, that's what most people call me. I am 63 years of age; married to my wife Christine for 37 years. We have three children and five lovely grandchildren. I was trained as an electrician and spent most of my adult life working for the British Government as an Electrical and Mechanical Supervisor, designing, building and maintaining military bases. I served in Hong Kong, Cyprus, Malta, Germany and, of course, in the UK where I spent 12 years working with the American Air Force on major airfields.

I participated in most sports and was generally quite fit although I was no Rambo!

I have IBM. On reflection, although I thought nothing of it at the time, I started to trip over things about 12 years ago (1988) and slowly but surely began to notice difficulties with grip, stair climbing and general all round motive power. This prompted me to visit my GP and culminated in my first appointment with a Neurologist and the first series of tests resulting in a diagnosis of Spinal Muscular Atrophy.

Nothing much happened for a couple of years until my physician became concerned that my symptoms were not following the SMA pattern and decided to arrange for a muscle biopsy. It was this test that determined that I had IBM and I was placed in the care of my current Consultant Neurologist.

Personally, I had never heard of IBM and apart from the consultant, I did not know anyone else who had, including my local GP. Thanks to IBMA and MAA I am now in contact with many people who do understand. My mission in life is to try to explain to anyone who asks and is willing to listen, just what IBM is and how it affects those unfortunate enough to get it.

I visit the Neurologist once a year, the Consultant Therapist as required and the home Occupational Therapist makes several visits each year to my home. ***I do not take any medication for IBM.*** This decision was made after discussion with my Neurologist and reading the results of various research surveys and the personal stories of individuals who have undergone a whole range of treatments. I have not seen or heard of any real proof that any of it actually works or has any beneficial effects.

I suppose the most traumatic period was the onset of falling, the instantaneous nature of which left me quite nonplussed and sometimes badly damaged, especially because these started quite early on and certainly before I was diagnosed with IBM. It would happen suddenly on the tennis court, whilst out walking or even just standing.

I have been a thespian for many years, musicals, light operetta, Gilbert & Sullivan, etc. so the most devastating moments of all were when my legs started to give out on stage when climbing or descending steps, etc., culminating in my having to give up this major part of my social life. I continued working until rising from a sitting position became too difficult and eventually a particularly nasty fall convinced me to apply for early medical retirement, which I did in March 1994.

Retirement has been far busier than I imagined. We have five grandchildren and I have been kept busy making doll houses, castles, etc., learning to play Bridge and, of course, the greatest time waster of them all - a computer!

We also belong to a small local Neurological Support Group which meets once a month for an informal chat and once a week for a Therapeutic swim.

Current, I am affected in both legs and arms, the left side being the worst. I wear calf/foot braces on both legs because of foot drop. Consequently, I dare not stand for long without the use of a wheeled frame and then only for transfers inside the house on flat carpeted floors by keeping my knees braced tightly together. Any relaxation results in a fall.

Hence, I find I spend a considerable amount of time in the wheelchair. This took me some time to come to terms with. (I didn't want people to think that I had given in without a fight!) But now, I'm a lot less tense and certainly feel more secure, knowing I'm not likely to finish up in an embarrassing heap on the floor! And additional bonus, according to Christine, is that it now takes only a fraction of the time to do the shopping!

Until recently, my car had hand controls, ultra light power steering, a thigh lifter which stands me up when getting out of the car and a small jib at the back to lift the electric wheelchair in and out. When we took delivery of the car, the independence it provided was like being set free and our quality of life improved tremendously. We now average 12,000 miles a year. Unfortunately, I have now had to give up driving due to increasing weakness in my arms. I rely on my long suffering wife to chauffeur me around. In May we take delivery of a specially converted Citroen "Berlingo" which will allow me access whilst staying in the wheelchair.

We have adapted the outside of the house by putting in wheelchair ramps, handrails and wide pathways, etc. My son is a Horticulturist and has altered the garden to be user friendly and easy to maintain.

My electric chair has a rising seat facility which makes me independent about the house. I have an electric recliner chair which also enables me to stand with a little help from Christine. The stair chair lift initially had the effect of turning our house into a bungalow so that no enforced move of home was necessary.

However, it eventually became too difficult for me to use and, of course, meant leaving my electric chair down stairs. It has now been replaced with the installation of a wheelchair through-the-floor lift which means I am now mobile upstairs and visit rooms I haven't seen in years!

We also have a bed capable of raising head and/or feet and a massage facility - wonderful! I need a mini portable hoist to enable Christine to transfer me from bed to chair/toilet. I have had considerable problems lately with numbness, mainly of lower legs and feet due to poor circulation. To try and alleviate this, I have now acquired a passive cycle exerciser which I can use whilst in the chair.

Lastly and probably the best piece of equipment for restoring dignity to one's life is a "Europa Electric Toilet Riser Seat."

All of the above have been acquired over a long period of time and I consider myself very fortunate, in conjunction with Social Services, to have been able to acquire them and make life a little easier. I mention them all only to give a more complete picture of my situation. If anyone would like details of any of the above, please do not hesitate to contact me.

There has been a lot of talk both locally and nationally about improving facilities for disabled people which at the current time in the UK are not too good. I did attend a local council meeting about three years ago, but whilst all the grandiose plans for the future sounded impressive, I was left with the fear that it all involved too many people forming too many committees. This proved an inevitably slowing of the process. This has since proved to be correct and for the last three years there have been plenty of meetings, but virtually no progress!

We were fortunate enough a few years ago while I could still manage it, to take a holiday to "Disney World" in Orlando, Florida and later a cruise on the Q.E. II and were impressed with the facilities provided for disabled people. I would be interested to know about the facilities in other areas. The holidays, by the way, were fantastic!

I enjoy reading the MAA "The Outlook" and especially look forward to the letters from members. We all have so many problems in common and it is great to read of the ingenuity and determination employed to overcome them.

I have recently become the European "Keep in Touch" (KIT) representative and am enjoying the challenge.

We are also fortunate to enjoy the close moral support of family and friends. Whilst we approach the future with a certain amount of trepidation, we are determined to get the most out of life as this restrictive condition will allow.

My best to all of you.

You may contact Bill at 113063.155@compuserve.com

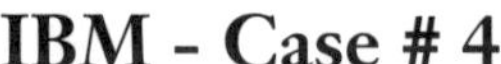

IBM - Case # 4

Diagnosed 1992 - Male
Present Age 73

Symptoms started in the 1970s with difficulty climbing stairs and falling when descending them. I fell off our pickup camper top several times. I tripped on 1/4" high places on ground when I was walking. I began to fall with no reason, even when holding on to something for solid support.

My present status: slowly progressing. Leg muscles and hand/finger muscles are very weak, but I can still walk a mile a day with a walker on level ground. I do not try to go up or down curbs or steps. I cannot rise from ordinary chairs, beds, or toilet seats. I use Ace bandage knee wraps whenever I leave the house. Now, I am also taking Methotrexate for medication if CPKs are normal. Looking back into the past, Prednisone I was prescribed several years ago probably caused me to get diabetes I can drive our minivan with accelerator pedal shaft lengthened. I cannot drive ordinary cars.

After my morning walk or an hour or so (1.3 mile) I am tired and rest most of the afternoon. I still do some aerobic exercises for arms and legs, but get too tired to do all the physician wants. Sciatica is a problem at times (IBM related?)

The way I've learned to live and cope with IBM is mostly being cautious and trying to maintain reasonable outlook on life. I have devices that look helpful; we have modified our home with 36" doors throughout, ramped (and bannistered where appropriate), all exterior doors, special flooring (linoleum type: no rugs), electric bed, hydraulic toil seat lift (Duette), canes placed everywhere.

I use a spring loaded riser seat in the dining room. Rubbermaid walker with seat and four wheels when walking or three wheeled scooter when distance is too great. We just purchased a Hoyer lift so my wife can lift me when I fall.

My wife is great! She is greatly concerned about me and is as helpful as she can be. I worry about what this stuff is during to her. Generally, we're doing pretty well; travel frequently (mostly by car - four round trips to the East Coast from California in two years.)

- Harry Johnson

IBM Case # 5

Diagnosed 1996
Female - Present Age 78

While spending part of the winter of 1995 in Florida with my sister and her husband, she prodded me to see a Neurologist because of weak arms and hands and the inability to rise easily from a low chair.

The search for a correct diagnosis continued in Colorado when I returned home. Dr. Smith did 52 blood tests and an EMG. His conclusion was that I had ALS. There was no way that this stubborn golf-playing lady would accept that diagnosis.

I asked for a second opinion and was referred to Dr. Steven Ringel, one of the top authorities on Neuromuscular diseases. A muscle biopsy cinched it! I will never forget that Dr. Ringel, a very busy man, called me at 8:30 on a Friday evening to ease my fears. He told me that I had IBM, not ALS.

I was prescribed that hellish drug Prednisone. It showed no improvement. After five months I stopped taking it. *No other drug or medication has been offered to me since then.*

To this day, my family does not realize how serious is IBM. They show some help when others are around, but let me fend for myself most times.

I have lost most of the use of my hands and my fingers will not bend. I played golf until I could no longer grip the club. I should have known there was a physical reason that my handicap skyrocketed. My dream was to play until the end of my time, but Fate saw it differently.

I am now 78 years old and can still walk a few feet. I manage with such helpful aids as two canes, a wheeled walker, an electric scooter, a recliner chair with a riser seat, risers on my bed to facilitate rising and a riser seat on the commode. There are many helpful assist bars around the shower and the commode. I wear a support elastic band on my left wrist so it doesn't flop around since all the controlling muscles are gone.

Perhaps the most embarrassing feature is my huge abdomen. Since all the muscles went bye-bye, my IBM is now attacking my large intestine and causing me to have a Spastic Colon.

I live in a Retirement Home. There is NO assisted living offered here. If my condition requires assistance, I will have to move elsewhere. I manage very well here, for the present, with the kind help of good friends. They help me with "buttons and bows" and a stair step here and there.

I play bridge two or three days weekly with the help of a card shuffler and card holder. When needed, my friends will deal for me.

I love to attend our Dallas Myositis Support Group luncheons and wish they were at least every other month. Jim Kilpatrick is a great organizer and Lucille, his wife, is so helpful and caring.

I did volunteer work in a school for one year. I had to give it up because of the low chairs - or spend the rest of my life in the hallway of Marcus Elementary School in Dallas.!

Now, I spend much time on my computer. When necessary, my son will install a Voice Activation on the computer for me.

My Email address is deecee@airmail.net.

Trusting that my tale isn't too boring, I remain,

Dee Charles, Dallas

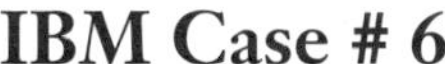

IBM Case # 6

Diagnosed 1997
Female

Hello! My name is Elisha. I am 38 years old and was diagnosed with IBM in the Spring of 1997, following tests, including a muscle biopsy. I don't know when my symptoms first started, . All I know is the first problem I noticed was much difficulty going up steps that didn't have handrails to hold on.

I thought this was be-cause I had gained too much weight too fast. I went from 130 pounds when I married in 1984 to near 200 pounds at times.

I had no pain and wouldn't have seen a doctor, but a nurse friend of mine saw me climbing the bleachers at the football game and thought that I had hurt my back! To get up steps without rails, I had to put my hand on my knee and push up as I take almost every step, or push on the seat part of the bleachers on the next row.

Anyway, I had told my nurse friend a few months prior how weak my leg muscles were and discussed it with her. After she saw me at the bleachers, she said that something was more wrong that just weak muscles, that I should see a doctor.

I went to our family doctor who did X-rays and an exam, but was not really sure what the problem was. She said maybe if I lost a little weight it would help. She also found almost no reflexes in my feet.

My family and friends advised that I should see a Neurologist and I did. First off, she was much larger than I and after she conducted the exam, she told me that she would bet me money that it was nothing to do with my weight. I wasn't really sure, but it did make me feel better! She even showed me how she didn't have those kind of problems getting out of chairs, up steps, or getting off the floor.

Flash forward a couple of months....

After many tests, she confirmed I had IBM! I had never heard of the disease. And she really didn't know much about it herself. My aunt got me some information from the Internet which helped tremendously.

At first, I was a little depressed, worried about things like if I would be able to help my daughters shop for wedding dresses when they get grown! Isn't it funny how that was the main thing I thought about as my daughters were only 9 and 11 at the time?

Anyway, I usually have a positive attitude and being a Christian, I believe that God allows everything to happen for a reason. My spirits lifted. I decided that I really had no pain like some people have every day. The only time I really hurt is when I've done shopping all day or work really hard physically.

Also, from what I read, it seems that IBM advances pretty slowly. I decided that I had a wonderful husband and two beautiful daughters so I wouldn't sit around feeling sorry for myself. I would do everything that I could, while I could!

Now, about three years later, I can't tell how much my IBM has progressed. I haven't been to the doctor since the fall of 1997 and still going strong. I haven't gone back to the doctor because it seemed there was really nothing for IBM. I would really like to talk to people who understand the problems I have. It's not that my family doesn't try to understand, but until someone finds out their body isn't "perfect," they can not fully understand how IBM affects a person.

I know I am not as bad as most, but there are still my "hard" things to face. One of the things that is really hard for me is lifting things off the floor. For instance, lifting a load of dirty clothes off the floor to take them from the bathroom into the laundry room. It seems so simple for most people, but I have to try to hold the clothes in one arm, and use the other to push up on the vanity to get up!

I can't even carry a bag of groceries up the steps to my door. I put them all on the porch, then go up and take them in one bag at a time.

Another thing is getting out of a chair while holding something, even as small as a baby, is very difficult, sometimes impossible, depending on the size and weight of the baby. Sometimes it seems that I lose my balance easily and I trip over nothing.

Well, I know this story is long, but I had been so excited about getting on the Internet and having a chance to talk with others, I just couldn't help myself!

I wish all of you well and I hope to hear from some of you.

- Elisha

jp2ebbaf@seark.net

IBM Case # 7

and Osteomyelitis, a bone infectious disease Diagnosed 1991 - Male Present Age 68

When the tailor charged $135 to weave a one inch slit in the knee of suit pants caused by another unexplained fall, it was time to find out the cause of the falls that were getting worse each time for the past several months.

I was scheduled to lead a group through Mexico. Because of my strength loss, pain and the uncertainty of all the testing being done, I continued the daily/weekly exams/testings with five specialists working as a group to find a diagnosis.

Without detailing the dozens and dozens of tests, in/out of hospitals, in/out of clinics, sessions with a sports surgeon, MRI's, EMG's; then, finally, the biopsy! IBM! The testing took three months.

After the Neurologist
met with my wife, son and me, she told me the only medication available that MIGHT help IBM was Prednisone.

Without hesitation, I told the physician that I would rather die than ever to be subjected to the curses of Prednisone again. I still feel that way.

In 1993, the doctor prescribed a spa to help with the pain and swelling in feet, ankles, and legs. The spa room adjoins my home office and I get into the spa often each day, depending on the pain.

Many mornings, I can barely get from my bed into the spa because of the pain, soreness and stiffness. What a blessed relief when the discomforts have vanished!

To this day, I have taken no medication for IBM.

*****

In 1995 I met with the original Neurologist for a comparative testing of the nerves and muscles with the 1991 tests. When I called the physician to make the appointment in 1995, the assistant told me I was the last person she ever expected with speak to again; asked who was taking care of my business and professional affairs, assuming I was in a nursing home as the neurologist had predicted in 1991.

In 1999 our HMO insisted that I have a complete round of testing with specialists outside our HMO. I know I have had tremendous strength loss without a $6,400 bill for a full examination to tell me what I already knew.

*****

When I was diagnosed August 9, 1991 and the Neurologist told me to have my professional responsibilities completed by the end of the year.

I was Comptroller of seven 501(c)(3) non profit organizations, a Board of Director member of seven corporations, and a professional organist.

I made immediate application in August for SSD and received the first payment in March 1992. Before the end of 1991 I was using a cane, had reduced my responsibilities. I had my "official" retirement March 8, 1992, being presented with a Proclamation from the Mayor, naming the day in my honor.

We had bought a large home about 80 miles Southeast of Dallas a couple years earlier in a little college town where we would eventually retire.

We lived in a Dallas town house that had five sets of stairs to climb to get to the bedrooms, baths and study. The large house was remodeled. No barriers.

By the end of 1991, I had moved into the house, living alone during the week. My son had moved furniture from the lake house and town house so I was comfortable and secure living alone My wife and son, both working in Dallas, came down on Friday evening and returned to Dallas Sunday evening.

At the 1991 diagnosis, the Neurologist prescribed a custom electric wheel chair I would be needing eventually. It took six months to be made but I don't use it (yet!). I had changed the cane for a quad cane, then to a walker. Insurance bought me a four wheel Pride Challenger scooter that I could use outside on the grounds, even going to the grocery store and visiting my mother in a nearby nursing home.
Because of the feet, legs and knees swelling and the intense

pain I had, the Neurologist prescribed medications that I have been taking since 1991 -

Motrin 800 mg 3x's daily
(as needed) for pain

Hydrocodone 5/500 mg (as needed for extreme severe pain)

Diazepam 10 mg (as needed to calm me after a fall)

Clonazepam 1 mg for the nightly leg cramps and spasms. Oh, how dreadful those things can be!

My physical condition at the present is loss of strength, can only walk a short distance with a walker, or balancing myself against the walls and furniture as I try to walk inside.

Our only son had assumed all the responsibilities of our properties, not worrying me about finances or any other problem that would stress or worry me. He and I were as close as any father and son.

*****

When I officially retired, I had completed 45 years as church organist (25 consecutive years on radio and television) and after the diagnosis and the move, I became organist for a local church which had purchased a new pipe organ with no one qualified to play it. My son took me to the church at 10:35 AM, meeting me again at 11:55 AM every Sunday.

All in all, my life was going well. I had made many new friends, still maintaining dinners with friends in Dallas, and being a certified Hospice counselor to AIDS patients in Dallas ten years, I volunteered again locally which lasted another 3 years.

*****

In November 1993 our 34-year old son died instantly with a massive heart attack as he returned from lunch; no warning, even though he had an full examination ten days before. I gave my son's eulogy. The eulogy was a promise to Rick I had made years before but never expected to have to fulfill.

Rick's death was de-vastating to me: his death, IBM, and the associated factors having to be faced and dealt with.

I am now taking Traza-done 50 mg daily, Doxapin 10 mg before eating. Later, I had to begin Zestril daily when my blood pressure became high.

*****

Besides IBM, an old bone infection disease - Osteomyelitis - resurfaced early May 1996 on my right lower leg.

I was in a Dallas hospital over two months, having six surgeries to keep the bone infection from reaching my blood stream which would poison my blood and kill me.

My wife was with me every day for 53 straight days at the hospital, without leaving because of my critical condition.

Because of the pain and heavy Morphine, I was un-conscious for six weeks. After the ambulance returned me home from Dallas, I had ten weeks in a hospital bed at home, three therapists, having to learn how to sit up, get up, stand up, to walk with the walker, then ultimately to drive my car again.

With the bone inflammation, I have to take Levaquin 500 mg/d for life in hopes of the infection never returning.

Because I had to be resuscitated three times after the sixth surgery, the physicians say I can not have any type of surgery.

We had sold the plane, our motor home, our son's boat and his trucks, but that hasn't stopped us from traveling. We divided our time between Florida and Texas for 2.5 years after our son's death.

(Prior to IBM, we had traveled abroad to several continents, the Far East, Mexico dozens of trips, the Islands and Hawaii.)

My daughter, son-in-law and two mid teen grandchildren, Lucille and I went on a cruise to the Caribbean islands and through the Panama Canal in 1998; and other trips into vacation areas in various states.

We attended the national conference of the MAA in Washington, D.C. in 1999.

We've been on several trips already this year (Branson, Mo.; Cincinnati, O.: and Pigeon Forge Tenn.) with more trips planned, going while we can.

*****

My involvements after IBM diagnosis, besides being an AIDS counselor for three years and organist locally for about a year, I stayed involved.

* I became a mentor at the local college to students with aca-

demic and music problems.

* I've used the ADA (Americans with Disabilities Act) laws well: signing a warranty for the arrest of the local mayor for using handicapped parking (*he WAS NOT reelected 10 days later when the newspaper ran the story on the front page two days.).*

* Using a Federal funding program available for this purpose, I filed Federal charges against two high rise office buildings' owners and management companies in Dallas for violations of the ADA. Two days before the Federal trial began, the buildings came into compliance, adding more handicapped parking spaces, lowering the door handles, slowing the elevator door's closing, release tension on exterior doors, rails at the commodes..

* In 1996, I began a Myositis Support Group in the Dallas area, the largest active group in the MAA organization, and have three Neurologists involved with our group who recommends our group to their Myositis patients. At this writing, a Houston Neurologist with several associates in four Neurological clinics are interested in involvement in our group, possibly making it a state wide Myositis support group.

At this writing, pro-sessional website specialists are designing a website for the support group. When activated, the Internet address will be www.MedicalSupportGroup.org.

Medical aids which have become necessary:.

* An electric four wheel heavy duty scooter

* An electric three wheel scooter with rear lift on my car to use in public away from home, shopping, dining, doctors, etc.

* The first electric wheel chair I got in used in the sun room.

* A three way electric
hospital bed with a trapeze head board for turning over and getting up. This was put into our home just prior to my return from the 1996 surgeries.

* A raised toilet

* An electric chair lift to help me stand

* Grabbers (the pointed and the suction cup types) for dozens of purposes.

I am able to walk few steps, using the wall and furniture to hold onto or using a walker. Thick carpets and re-finished parquet floors make me lose my balance easily. Losing our balance seems to be a problem with most IBM patients.

I am still able to shower, shave, dress myself without help. (I cannot wear dress shoes with strings, because my feet swell too often. Also, the soles of all shoes have to be ribbed, not plain leather soles.) Driving my car is no problem for me on the recent 2,500 mile trip - just adjusting the seat like a La-Z-Boy and enjoy the scenery!

I have a regular home business office, fully equipped for my work. I work virtually all day at my desk and computer, raising my feet and legs often.

Being an avid reader, to relax, I take two morning papers, and read various subjects. I just finished reading the downfall of the Roman Empire during the leadership of the various Emperors.

In 1999 I supplied various Myositis materials to 46 patients who had contacted me, by phone or E-mail, referred to me from the MAA offices, seeking help getting SSD or specific Myositis literature.

*****

I've had my share of bleeding knees, elbows and hands, even a slice in my scalp that required the ER and six staples put into my scalp.

Without the help and support of my dear wife of 47 years, I couldn't have made it alone. She recognizes when I am too weak to accept social commitments so there's no argument.

Whenever I get up and make my bed and dressed, she knows I'll be alright through the day. Those few days when I try to get out of bed, but just don't have the strength, she understands and shields me from calls and visitors.

We have household and lawn care help since we can't do it now.

In addition to my IBM and Osteomilitis problems to deal with, my mother is in a nursing home a few blocks from our home in the last stages of Alzheimer's. She is 85 years old. Lucille checks on her often, but I don't go often now.

When I have been extremely tired, two or three nights I will sleep 12 to13 hours straight each night. On a recent long trip, two nights I slept 16 hours without waking.

We eat dinner in Dallas with our daughter and family often. I also have lunch or dinner with my friends often. We drive once or twice a weekly to Dallas for dining, seeing physicians, banking or business purposes.

Lucille is on the Executive Auxiliary Board of the local hospital and works two days a week at the church's family life center office. She's in the choir and I encourage her to take the Senior trips out of town often for a few days, knowing she also needs a change and I am content and secure being in my home "comfort zones.".

Whether men realize it or not, the women are not the weaker sex! Those of us with IBM know this without question!

IBM Case # 8

Diagnosed Oct. 1997
Male - Present Age 74

I have Inclusion Body Myositis. I am a male, 74 years old. My correct diagnoses was given in October 1997. However, my first diagnoses was given in February 1992.

I don't know when the first symptoms of the muscle disease started, but would venture to say it was in the 1980's. I was having problems climbing stairs as well as descending them. At times when walking, my knees would buckle underneath me and I always fell backwards, never forward. That did make me wonder!

I had a heart attack in January 1991 and received five bypasses. Walking became a big part of my rehabilitation program. I eventually was able to walk 2.5 miles each day. I fell one day in my home after returning from my work, struck my head on the stationary bicycle pedal that required some stitches

Our family physician asked how it happened and I explained it to him, then told him I had been falling from time to time because my legs would buckle under me. I have difficulty getting up from the falls. He thought since I am a diabetic, perhaps my nerve signals were not working too well. He suggested I see a Neurologist to have some tests done.

After my first visit to the Neurologist, he told me, after completing the usual tests, "I believe you have a muscle disease." To be certain, there were more testing to be done and a trip to the hospital. It was February 1992. I had two muscle biopsies: the first was from my right upper arm. The second from my right upper thigh.

The laboratory, where the tissue was sent, gave a diagnoses of Polymyositis. The Neurologist gave me some exercises to do. He said, 'If you don't do these each day, the wheel chair waits at the end of the hall."

Before leaving the hospital, I was on an IV drip of Solumedrol. Then on discharge day, a prescription for Prednisone, 10 mg, three times a day. My wife and I left in a daze, no additional information or facts were given to use about this disease.

I did the exercises, continue to work as often as I could, and continued to grow weaker. I had to have my wife help me rise from any sitting position. She did this by pulling me up front by belt loops in the back of my pants.

In the next six months following the missed diagnoses, I was even more weaker. When I visited my doctor, why wasn't the exercise working for me? He suggested I go into Rehab for awhile. So, I dd. I had more IV Solumedrol and was fitted for knee braces.

Never once was I told anything about Polymyositis. Seven weeks later I was placed in Out-Patient Therapy. There I had an indoor pool for exercises for the next three months. Muscle strengthened my arms and legs. I continued until fall and grew very concerned as why nothing was really helping me!

Being a diabetic, taking Insulin, the steroids through my blood sugars went out of sight and it required me to take even more Insulin to keep it under control. This was frustrating to no end. My life seemed totally out of my control. I wondered when, where, this muscle disease was taking me.

It was at this time I started walking with one cane, then before long, two canes. I still had terrible falls. My hands were losing their strength, fingers were not always able to retrieve things I needed picked up. I became an angry, frustrated "Man" as it seemed. I was losing all of my abilities I once had.

For five years I was to believe Polymyositis was my disease; and I hated her as she caused me to fall every where I went, and mostly because I no longer had any control over my own body.

In May of 1997, I suffered a terrible fall. It was the one that finally led me to where I am today. I was trying to open a door, in a public restroom. It was too hard for me even using two hands. My feet began sliding and I did the splits! I fell to the tile floor with my right leg bent under me and the other leg in the opposite direction. I was alone in this room and down on the floor for ten minutes.

My wife came to see why I hadn't returned to our table where we were eating lunch. When help finally came, I could not stand on my right leg. They put me in a dining room chair and carried me to my car. When we arrived home, my wife couldn't get me out of the car. She took me to the emergency room and was X-rayed from hip to below the knee. No broken bones, but a very bad hamstring puffed muscle.

I was due to have another biopsy in two days. It was decided to just keep me in the hospital until that time. Then I had the third biopsy on the side of my right thigh. The surgeon said he found no muscle tissue left in my thigh, only chopped fat. What muscle you lose, you never regain.

Ten days I spent in the hospital before the Neurologist said, "You can go home with a wheel chair today." I told him, "No, not today!" He had me transferred again to the Rehab hospital for seven weeks where once again I had more IVs of Solumedrol. After a few more days this began to cause me pain in my stomach. I no longer was able to use the Solumedrol. I was fitted for new leg braces, given more exercises, and six weeks later I was dismissed, with the doctor telling my family they should begin looking for a nursing facility as my wife would not be able to care for me longer than two years!

I was dismissed on July 3, 1997 with my new wheel chair, walker, reacher, a dressing hook, a bath bench, and portable bedside commode! And I didn't want ANY of them. I also had a Home Health Service to help us for one year. It was through them that I was led to Muscular Dystrophy Association where I finally received some clue about Polymyositis.

They asked if I needed any help. I said, "I think I may need some help." They gave me an appointment in September 1997. I had my medical records forwarded to them.

The Neurologist looked at me and said, 'I scanned your records and I did not see how you absolutely could have Polymyositis. It may look like possible Polymyositis, but I don't believe you have it. I think you have IBM."

The Neurologist explained all that to us. Then he asked for another muscle biopsy and I agreed to have it - #4 biopsy taken from my left arm muscle. It was sent to the wrong lab and by the time it got to the right lab, there was not enough live tissue left.

So... I returned three weeks later and had # 5 biopsy - and it turned out to be the FINAL BIOPSY! The report came back. Without a doubt I had Inclusion Body Myositis. There was no treatment for this muscle disorder. The doctor said, 'No one should have had to have five muscle biopsies to find out what muscle disease you have." At last, my family and knew what I had.

My wife is my care giver and she is still able to take care of me. I am wheel chair bound and find I need all the equipment I could get after all. My wife uses a gait belt, her body and her strength, to pull me up to the walker and I can walk a short distance to the bathroom.

I also have an electric Rascal power chair with a joy-stick control. The seat of the chair can raise me six inches to assist me when I need to be higher. We have a minivan with a companion seat power mechanical switch which will turn out toward the open door and move out the door and tilt down so she can transfer me into the van seat. The seat is returned inside the van, move a lever, and re-turn me toward the front of the van. This makes for pure enjoyment. It is easy for both of us!

NO! I don't like IBM either "as it is not nice to it's host!" I, along with all the other IBMers, must wait, must hope and must pray each day when we will get a call telling us, "Come in. We at last have found a treatment and cure for you!"

IBM Case # 9

Diagnosed 1996 - Male Present Age 88

Can't - Just a few short years ago that word was not in my vocabulary. Now I have used it to change many things in my lifestyle. I am a male, born in Texas in 1912.

Because of falling several times in 1991, I felt that my left knee was giving me trouble. My doctor referred me to an Orthopedic surgeon. After a CAT scan and a MRI, we discovered a torn cartilage. Arthroscopic surgery removed the torn cartilage, but I was still subject to frequent falls.

I was then referred to a Neurologist. We tried to determine the cause of the torn cartilage - I am, or was, an avid horseman and we thought that while getting on and off a horse that the left leg was used to support the entire weight of the rider and twisted the foot 90 degrees.

In 1993 I had a muscle biopsy on the right hip and was diagnosed with Polymyositis. At that time, the doctor prescribed 65 mg/day Prednisone. Shortly after taking the Prednisone, I had a very severe diarrhea problem that hospitalized me for several days. No one would admit that the Prednisone caused this, but I think it did. However, my body finally adjusted.

In 1996 I had another muscle biopsy. This time it was on the left hip and was diagnosed as Inclusion Body Myositis (IBM). Prednisone was continued at a tapering rate of 2 and one-half mg every other day until September 21, 1999.

Today, all that I take is 1500 mg Calcium+D and a One-a-Day vitamin - and, of course, Tylenol!

I had an infusion of immunoglobulin at a rate of 500 mg/day for five consecutive days. No change was observed. At the request of the Neurologist, I started physical therapy on a limited basis. It was then I made the profound statement that if God wanted me to touch my toes, He would have put them on my knees!

My use of mechanical aids started in 1992 with the use of a cane. I am constantly looking for aids to make me as mobile as possible. For ex-ample, there is one step going into our den where I have fallen several times. At my wife's insistence, we had hand grab bars installed on each side of the door and designed a wedge so that I can walk up the step in an easy manner. When invited to visit friends, we have to drive by their home to make sure that we can manage the steps. (Don't count on others to say there are no steps!)

I have purchased every aid I can find, including two canes, two walkers, two La-Z- Boy electric lift chairs, high rise lift attachment to fit in my dining chair and every time I need help to get up, we just add another pillow to the seat!

There are hand rails by the bed as well as both sides of the hall. I have had a high-rise toilet seat added as well as louvered bathroom doors that open outward.

Can't hasn't stopped me yet for doing all that I am able to do with IBM.

(Later, this delightful couple purchased a beauty- barber shop chair to use at the dining room table.)

IBM Case # 10

Diagnosed 1976
Female - Present Age 82

The year was 1976. My leg pains were diagnosed as Polymyositis with the help of a biopsy in each leg.

For three years before this, I was treated for arthritis, mainly with aspirin, which had no more effect than a drink of water.

Finally, my legs refused to take even a step.. I spent a month in the hospital and the medication prescribed was 800 mg/day Prednisone.

There were two years of physical therapy and CPK blood tests every three months. The dosage of Prednisone was regulated according to the CPK tests. The side effects of Prednisone are too numerous to mention, including several surgeries.

Finally, I was able to walk without help for a few years. It wasn't long before I couldn't rise from a seated position without pushing up on armrests and the use of a cane. Also, speech and hand therapies were necessary. For the hand therapy, I was given paraffin tank and exercises to do for my stiffening hands.

Then the falling started. (I still remember the first time at the local shopping mall). At first, I only fell down, landing in a sitting position, and then I started falling straight backwards. (I guess I have a hard head, because it never cracked!) This called for a series of MRI's to check for a brain tumor. After that was eliminated, it was decided that I was having mini-strokes (TIA). I still do not believe that this was true. After all this, the worst pain was yet to come which was give up driving my car in 1986. (No mind and leg coordination.)

Twice, the CPK went down low enough to stop Prednisone. Soon all the old problems came back and so Prednisone was started again.

In 1995, I had a mastectomy. It has not spread after five years. (One of the lucky ones!)

Finally, in 1997, the percentages caught up with me. Thirteen days after my husband of fifty-six years died, I fell and broke my hip. It healed fine.

Prior to this, I had used a walker for several years and in 1994 I bought a scooter for the long haul. However, a year ago, I was forced to use a wheel chair all the time, inside and outside.

At the age of 82, it seems I will have yet another diagnosis. It is IBM. At the first Myositis Support Group in Dallas, begun and led by James Kilpatrick, I ever attended, I asked the speaker what was happening to my hands. He said, "You have IBM." MDA clinic examined me and said I had all the signs of IBM. However, a biopsy must be had to definitely confirm this. At this time, I have not yet decided on this procedure.

I am still on 5 mg/day Prednisone and have been for the last three years and I have a fear of what might happen if I stop Prednisone.

Recently, I have experienced "foot drop" and plan to see a physical medicine doctor about braces; if they will help.

After all this, I am thankful to still have a sound mind. The only memory loss I have had has been word recall. In that case, I beat around the bush until the brain cells connect.

Throughout the progress of the disease, I had complete support and understanding from my family. It is harder to deal with now that I am alone and the depression is more prevalent.

At the onset of my disability, I felt guilty for not being able to carry on my usual activities and duties. One of the most frustrating aspects of Myositis is that your looks are deceiving in the sense that your looks do not portray your disability.

Along the way, I learned a few tricks to help me to cope, as follows:

* A rack that extends over the full width of the end of the bed made with PVC keeps the covers off my burning, aching feet.

* I put tiny balloons on lamp switches for friction.

* Non-sterile surgical gloves help for anything that needs friction to handle.

* Telescoping metal back scratchers (from 6.5" to 26") besides scratching your back, are good for turning off/on wall switches and pick up items that just seem to float out of your hands.

* I have the postman place mail in a plastic basket by the door and I just open the door and drag it in with my scratcher.

* I also have Dysphagia and use orange "Chill" to help swallow numerous pills. (I have had the procedure to lessen this problem and it has helped.)

At the present time, I am able to live alone with the daily assistance of a young lady. However, I am considering moving to a new retirement residence in my local community to eliminate the responsibility of maintaining a house. When I can no longer perform basic activities of daily living, I will be forced to move to assisted living.

Hopefully, I will always be able to manage for myself for many more years.

IBM Case # 11

Diagnosed June 1997
Female - Present Age 81

In June of 1997 I was admitted as a patient to the Mayo Clinic in Rochester, MN where I was diagnosed as having IBM. For 77 years I had been very healthy with no major illnesses that might have depleted my strength. However, in 1994 I noticed I was losing strength in my legs and I could not attribute the disability to any known reason. I knew something was wrong.

Because climbing stairs was becoming more and more difficult, plus falling often, my local doctor referred me to a Neurologist who diagnosed my condition as "Lou Gehrig's Disease" (ALS).

Since I did not exhibit many of the other symptoms of ALS, I felt a more adequate analysis would be available through the Mayo Clinic.

At the Mayo Clinic I underwent over 40 tests and IBM showed up in one of the muscle tests. They indicated there was no method of treatment available they were aware of, but the disease would probably progress very slowly.

Since my Grandmother had died with "Parkinson's Disease," I asked the doctors at Mayo if IBM was also hereditary. They said no, that this was an immune system disorder disease and not hereditary. (I personally believe that the opposite is true; that it is a hereditary disease.) Therefore, the disease did progress slowly for about a year, but then, suddenly, progressing rapidly, causing complete disability within the next year and a half.

My local doctor prescribed Methotrexate and Folic Acid, which I have been taking for over a year, but the progress of the disease has not been altered. I continue to lose muscle mass as muscle deterioration increases.

At this time, I am unable to stand without the aid of something to hold onto, walk without a walker, or do any type of housework. I am able to get around the house in a wheel chair or on a scooter. Luckily, the scooter will go through all the doors in the house and I can ride the scooter outside in the yard.

I am thankful there has been minimum pain associated with my particular case of IBM. I feel well and do not feel comfortable complaining because I see the condition of others with this disease who are in much more discomfort than I have experienced.

Most of all, I am thankful for my husband, Fuller, who is my caregiver and provides my every need.

- Elizabeth Mason
Henderson, Texas

IBM Case # 12

Diagnosed 1982 - Male
Present Age 75

I am a 75 year old male with IBM or the *BIG BLUE* as I call it. I was misdiagnosed as having Myositis in 1982. I had an upper thigh biopsy and it was still called Myositis.

Prednisone was prescribed and I took as much as 20 mg/day for pains in the knees and elbows. It was reduced, but I couldn't take less than 5 mg/day or the pain came back.

To offset the Prednisone, I also took Slow K but that was not until 1987.

I started to wear compression hose to reduce the swelling in my legs. I began Methotrexate in October 1987 and took it until September 1988. It did not work, so I stopped taking it. I kept on with the Prednisone and wore straps around my knees. They helped very much.

In 1990 I started with the Muscular Dystrophy Association. The doctors there kept me on the Prednisone and Slow K 600 mg. In September 1989 I had a biopsy of the upper left arm and only then was told that I had Inclusion Body Myositis (IBM). I also had Magnetic Resonance Imagining (MRI) done and was shown the dead muscles and also those that were still active.

I was still taking Prednisone and Slow K.

I have had pneumonia three times and now can tell when it is coming again. I also have trouble swallowing or Dysphagia, as it is called.

When at the first I started falling, I started using a cane. That was in 1982 and then in 1987 I started using a walker, then in 1990 to 1993, it was a three wheeler and then into an electric wheel chair (Love Lift). It was called that because it had a feature that went up and down, which made it easier for me to stand. I cannot stand now.

I have no use of my left hand but with massage therapy, I can use my right hand. I also feed myself with the use of a feeder arm attached to my wheelchair.

I have never asked, "Why me?" You accept the disease and its progression, but the disease itself will never kill me. You just do not give up! Continue fighting day by day.

I think the person and his care giver must always keep an open mind and be inventive as to how to make things easier, such as wide rubber bands on taps and door handles, extended straws (high pressure auto-motive tubing), wooden levers for opening car doors and cupboards, soap on a rope, and a hanging container suspended from the ceiling for drinks while sitting in a lift chair.

In 1998 I moved from Texas to the Veterans Hospital in Canada because my care giver was no longer able to help physically. Now, I keep very busy with new projects, thanks to the help of many therapists at the hospital.

(Editor's note: This gentleman began water coloring painting. He has won several ribbons for his art. His paintings are hung in the hallways of the VA Hospital. When they lived in Dallas he had never painted before.)

IBM Case # 13

Diagnosed 1996
Female - Present Age 70

My name is Bobbye Finley. I am a 70 year old female who was diagnosed with Inclusion Body Myositis in 1996.

I was teaching second grade in Tyler, Texas in 1993, when I began to notice some medical problems that seemed very strange to me.

I experienced several unexplained falls. My knees were very weak and would often just give way. Fortunately, there were no serious injuries as a result of these falls.

Another problem that plagued me was the failure to rise from a sitting position. My strength seems to disappear and waves of weakness came over me. I had always been very active, but now I had to restrict my actions. I soon resorted to setting on a tall stool to help me fulfill my responsibilities to my students.

These problems continued after I retired in May 1994. In fact, they became so severe that I sought medical attention many times from my family physician. He was unable to provide a solution, so he referred me to a Tyler Neurologist. The Neurologist conducted several tests, but he did not feel confident with his findings. He, then, made arrangements for me to see the Neurologists at the University of Texas Southwestern Medical Center in Dallas, Texas.

At this time the realization that this was no ordinary ailment began to dawn on me. Although I dreaded finding out what was going on in my body, I was determined to pursue any chance of improvement and, hopefully, recovery.

On December 2, 1996 three Neurologists at UT Southwestern Medical Center agreed that I had a chronic disease called Inclusion Body Myositis. They shared the information there was no known treatment or cure for IBM.

They prescribed Presdnisone for the pain I was experiencing. The dosage was quite high but I managed to endure the side effects for a few months. The pain level was reduced and my CK level also was lowered. However, as soon as the dosage was lessened, the pain returned and my CK level rose.

In May 1999, I began to participate in a study to determine the effect of Beta Interferon on the disease. I concluded the treatments in November 1999. The results of this study have not been released at this time.

At the present time, I am receiving no medication except for pain killers, which manage my pain fairly well.

To prevent falling, I use a rolling walker that permits me to sit if I begin to tire. My activities have been severely curtailed. Cooking and cleaning have become difficult to accomplish. Climbing steps has become an almost impossible task. The weakness in my arms, hips, and legs is my major problem. I have also experienced some difficulty in swallowing.

I join with my dear friends who also suffer with this disease in hoping and searching for a treatment and cure to aid our recovery. MAY IT COME SOON!

IB2M Case # 14

Male - Inherited IBM

My story of IBM is hard for me to write since it also the story of my mother who I lost to the consequences of IBM.

I have IBM, probably one of the first to be diagnosed as

inheriting the disease. I first recognized the symptoms in 1986 (a feeling of off balance while running and difficulty in rising from a stooped position.)

Looking back, however, I remember that I have always had weak ankles which resulted in many painful falls (this goes back to my late 20's before IBM was known.)

There has been a very slow, steady wasting of both my proximal and distal muscles, but until very recently, I have been completely independent.

My condition at this time is at it's worst. I cannot make a fist with my left hand. I cannot make a muscle with my left arm; both quads are gone; I cannot move my left toes, but I am still mobile.

I have a three wheel scooter that gets me where I want to go. I have raised my bed and my La-Z-Boy about 4 inches to aid access both in and out.

So far, my investment on special needs items have been limited to a 17" rise toilet and hand rails, the 3 wheeled walker, cane and wheel chair that were my mothers. Thank God, I haven't had to use the wheel chair yet.

I am now dealing with one of the most serious symptoms (in my opinion) of IBM, "Dysphagia," the difficulty in swallowing. This is the condition that led to my mother's death. I will not go into the details here, but if anyone is interested, you can reach me through James R. Kilpatrick's email or his home address.

IBM Case # 15

Male
"Coping with IBM"

In response to my experience with IBM, I will start about 8 or 9 years ago. I would go to doctors for different aches, pains and falling down. When I came in from work, I used to get out and walk in the evening for my exercise.

One day when I was walking, my left leg just folded under me and I fell. When I was walking 2 or 3 weeks later, my right leg would fold. Again, some 6 months would go by before I would fall again, usually always when I was taking my walks.

I didn't think too much about it at the time I was getting to the age when arthritis or bursitis could be a factor. The doctors could not find anything wrong. They would just speculate on different things.

Then, as more time passes, I would notice when I would try to get off the couch or chair, I would have to use my hands and arms to help push me up. At the time, I still was not thinking too much about it, because I did not have to do that all the time.

As time continued to pass, I noticed I would have to "push" up more and more. When I was on the commode, I would have to push, using the vanity and tub. At the dining table, I would use the table to push up.

I continued to work and go through my daily routine. I got by decently. But I knew something was wrong somewhere, but the doctors still could not find anything wrong. I went through this for several years.

In January 1997 while living in Florida, I went to a doctor that hooked me up to a machine and stuck needles into my muscles, He said, "Mr. Christian, I don't know what is wrong with you and I don't have a diagnosis to tell you, but you definitely have something seriously wrong with you because this machine is going crazy. If I were you, I would go to my family doctor and have him order a muscle biopsy."

So, that is what I did.

The procedure was ordered and I went into the hospital for the muscle biopsy. The doctor went into my thigh where my biggest muscle was cut about a 4" slit. A large piece of muscle was removed and sent to the lab for testing. The result was INCLUSION BODY MYOSITIS.

The surgeon explained what IBM was. "At this time, it is a terminal disease with no treatment." My family doctor had not heard of it before. My family started to do research to see more about what it was and how to treat it. Were there special diets, treatments, exercise or medications?

No one seemed to have answers. We got information off the Internet that helped explain what IBM was. I wrote the Myositis Association of America and got information with names of people who had different varieties of Myositis.

We wrote letters to the 32 people in our region in Florida. We asked them about their experience with Myositis. We asked what doctors they used, what exercise they did, what medication did they take, if any, and what did they recommend.

Out of the 32 letters we mailed, we got 30 responses very soon. Some were letters and some by phone.

"We know what you want to hear that 'Yes, there is something that will help or something that you can do or take. We are sorry to say there is nothing that will help. There is no cure. There is no medication that has proven to be safe and really helpful for IBM. Some have tried some recommended medications but it has not been helpful.'"

It burst my bubble. I was looking for someone to come up with a solution for me and this disease.

My doctor I had used several years contacted the University of Florida - a Tampa Medical School. We thought we might get a second opinion. He talked with a medical professor that knew about IBM. That doctor said if I had been diagnosed with IBM, that was it and that is what it was.

With the symptoms and the biopsy results, there was no need to do a second biopsy; the results being the same. He told me to keep in contact with MAA as they might know of some changes that would be forthcoming. He urged me to keep searching on my own for additional information.

Over a period of time, I was not using assistance of any kind to get around. I began to use a cane, but I needed something else in a short period of time. I was told to get a walker, but my pride was in the way and I didn't want to use a walker so I began using two canes. This worked for about a year. Finally, I got to the point I had to give in and use a walker.

In addition, it was hard to get on and off my bed. We tried something to help. We got PVC pipe what was the same size of the bed legs, cut the pipe to length I needed and put them under the bed legs to raise the bed to be higher. We put caps on the bottom of each leg. I was able to get into and out of the bed much easier.

At this point, we moved to Texas to be closer to our children for their physical support. I continued using the walker only. Afraid of getting outside with just the walker because my legs had gotten weaker and weaker, I got a scooter for travel outside the house.

To this day, I still use my scooter as my car to move about outside. I now have an electric wheel chair and lift chair. I depend on these very heavily. We purchased a van equipped with a lift for the scooter. I did not drive anymore. This is my way of getting out and away from the house for awhile. Usually, my wife or one of the three children are able to do the driving. They drive me to the doctor, dentist or just driving around for recreation. I do not travel a lot because of the equipment I need every day at home.

In December 1999 I had the Endoscopy and Esophageal Dilation. I had gotten some information from others with the same problem in swallowing. For me, the procedure did not work. I still have problems swallowing. The doctor said if there was some obstruction in the esophagus then stretching it would probably help. I did not have any obstruction so guess that was the main reason the procedure didn't help me.

I have been very lucky to have medical insurance. I have acquired most of my equipment through the in-surance. This has helped tremendously. We bought another inner spring mattress to add to the one on the bed. This raised the bed higher as I needed it to get on and off the bed easier.

With my three children, I have been lucky as they are always available to help in whatever needs to be built or remodeled that will help me in what need I have each day.

Other small things can be a help. One day I was having so much trouble cutting my fingernails. I would lose grip of the clippers or drop them. It would take me hours and several tries to get my nails cut. I decided to try something. Using packaging tape, taping the clippers to a table top. Now, I can do my nails in about 15 minutes with ease.

With IBM we try to invent items to make our lives easier. Another problem is unscrewing containers like jars and bottles. If anyone has an answer to this, let me know.

Today is March 25, 2000. As of this date, I do not have answers to the IBM questions. In the course of this disease, I have discovered "Quest Magazine" from the Muscular Dystrophy Association which contains lots of good articles. There is information concerning "Helps" with medical equipment. I have ordered several items that have helped me very much. One item was a commode riser that lifts the commode off the floor 6 inches. And it looks nice.

I have been blessed with my three children and wife of 42 years. She has been by my side through everything. That has probably been the greatest asset I have. To have someone who cares for you and you are cared for is a blessing. The hardest thing I have had to do is to keep a positive mental attitude and to strive to keep plugging. If the good Lord lets me live long enough, I will master that as well.

Any suggestions would be welcomed.

You can E-mail us at BCRLC@juno.com.

- Ronald Christian

Sanger, Texas.

IBM Case # 16

Male - Present Age 68
Inclusion Body Myositis Case Report

As a former YMCA summer camp executive director, I averaged six miles a day of walking. I retired in 1991 after 25 years. Life has changed somewhat since then, but not as badly as I had heard.

I discovered I had a left foot drag about 1986 when I was 54 years old, the age range for males who might get IBM. Because of a very alert Neuro-logist in Vermont, I received necessary tests and a muscle biopsy.

Since there's no known cause or cure, he prescribed vitamins as therapy of 1000 IU of Vitamin E and 100 mg of Vitamin B Complex each day. I have continued that routine and have not taken any medications for IBM.

I was fitted for a plastic below-the-knee brace for the left leg about four years ago. I also got one for the right leg. My distal muscles have atrophied so much I can not do steps and I use a cane to help with my balance.

I have not allowed IBM to interfere with the quality of my life. We live in a one floor apartment so there are no steps except outside to the street level. I walk my dog four times a day. I swim three days a week and play in four different bands with weekly rehearsals and many concerts. Also, I volunteer at a desk at our local hospital eight hours a week.

I have no pain related to IBM so I am very lucky. My wife and I travel on out of town trips five or six times a year. We attend theater, concerts and movies regularly, using elevators when necessary and getting seats on the first level.

While my muscles have obviously weakened a little more each year, I am optimistic of living a fairly long and normal life as long as I take care to avoid falls, which do happen while walking my dog.

Swimming is excellent exercise for IBM patients, but it must be kept to a regular schedule to be beneficial.

I expect to see no cure and only limited treatments. Many IBM patients are worse off than I. I am grateful to be spared pain.

- Robert V. Sanders Virginia

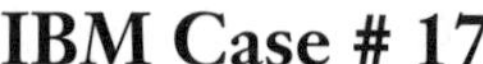

IBM Case # 17

Diagnosed PM 1990
Diagnosed IBM - Jan. 2000
Female - Present Age 69

Hi, everyone:

My name is Mary Walsh. I am 69 years old. I was first diagnosed as having PM by a top Rheumatologist at a top hospital about ten years ago. I was prescribed Prednisone 10 mg/d for most of that time.

In January 2000, my diagnoses was changed to IBM. In the previous 10 years it was never even suggested that I needed to have a muscle biopsy. If it had been suggested, I would have had one immediately.

When other tests suggested that the muscles were turning to fat, my doctor suggested a Neurologist to examine me. The Neurologist immediately felt I did not have PM, but perhaps an adult form of Muscular Dystrophy. I was quite concerned because MD, of course, is genetic. I was worried about my children and grandchildren.

The Neurologist suggested that a biopsy was needed. I had the muscle biopsy and the results came back showing a definite diagnosis of IBM. I was angry that I had been taking Prednisone unnecessarily for so many years. Now, I am trying to wean myself off Prednisone.

Approximately for 20 years or so I have done water exercises 3 or 4 times a week which were of great benefit to me both physically and mentally.

I was extremely active and an independent person. I am now attempting to humble myself because I often need help getting out of a chair or seat, often a stranger will see me struggling and will help me.

The most difficult aspect of this malady for me is accepting help from anyone. It is painful for me as I am used to doing for others.

I have been fortunate with this disease, also. It has certainly been slow moving into my body. I can actually trace my weakness back about 23 years. Trouble getting on a bus, rising from a crouched position, etc.

I feel that the absence of "hope" with IBM is difficult. Knowing there is no cure or even treatment is quite overwhelming.

About 11 years ago, before I was diagnosed with the disease, I took out a long term nursing care insurance policy, because, I knew that I was not as strong as other women my age. I thank God I did this. I would never want to live with my children, even though they are extremely good to me.

The things I miss most - walking on the beach, or even sitting on the beach, being able to walk to concerts and shows, being more active with my grandchildren, going on bus trips or traveling.

But I am grateful for the many good years I have had and the many activities I took part in before this disease took over my body.

- Mary Walsh

IBM Case # 18

Diagnosed PM 1983, Diagnosed IBM 1993
Male - Present Age 69

I am a 69-year-old male living in Southwest Virginia. I first became aware of weakness in my legs about 25 years ago. I went to a general practitioner and received no help except to exercise more. I continued to lose strength and went to an Internist in 1983 where I was diagnosed with Polymyositis after undergoing a biopsy at the University of Virginia.

I was prescribed Methotrexate and Prednisone which were given to me in various doses over a period of years. I continued to lose strength in my arms and legs until I was unable to get up from a normal chair and was subject to falling in which I have suffered minor bruises and broken bones.

I went to NIH in 1993 to participate in a Polymyositis study. The NIH physicians changed my diagnosis to IBM because I had been given a biopsy previous to going to the hospital and they found most fat cells in my muscles and were not able to get enough muscle tissue for a biopsy.

In 1997, I received IVIg through Dr. John Armstrong at Selma Medical Clinic in Winchester, Virginia. I received five days of treatment per week for four months. I did not notice any significant benefit following the treatment, but my condition had seemed to stabilize and I have not lost any strength since then.

I cannot go up or down stairs or step over curbs, but I am

still able to walk using mechanical assistance. My neighbors built a ramp which enables me to get in and our of the house without difficulty.

* I installed a stair lift in my home which allows me complete access to any part of my home.

* I bought a used minivan which has high seats so I can get out of the van and still be able to drive.

* I have raised my bed on blocks and have put blocks under the chairs I use in the home.

* I have raised my bathroom commode to 24 inches by using a bedside commode.

* I have a walker with two wheels which I use inside my home and a four-wheel walker which I use when I go to a restaurant or shopping.

My wife and daughter assist me greatly when I need assistance in standing when I do things outside my home.

I am now on Prednisone 15 mg every other day and Methotrexate 15 mg once a week. I have diabetes which is made worse by the Prednisone. I also take over the counter supplements consisting of COQ10, Creatine, a-lipoid acid, and a multivitamin. I attempted to take the L-Carnitine but suffered severe diarrhea and was forced to stop.

As I stated before, the IVIg treatments have stabilized my condition and I have seemed to gain some strength. I also will continue taking the health supplements as long as I remain in this stable condition.

I was employed as a CPA and was able to work until I was 65 years old because the work did not require physical activity, although I did have difficulty in getting in and out of client offices by the time of my retirement.

- B. J. Roanoke, Va.

IBM Case # 19

Diagnosed March 1995
Male - Age 78

To those who may have contracted IBM or another type of Myositis, I hope my experience may be helpful in coping with this oddball condition.

In retrospect, my symptoms began several years ago. On occasion I would have difficulty walking, especially knee movements. Since the problems weren't permanent, I had no idea I had a condition that would lead to Myositis

My condition was diagnosed in March 1995. I became very unsteady on my feet and I was falling without any reason.

My Neurologist had tests run to check my strength and nerve reactions. The most convincing evidence was a biopsy on the muscle of my thigh.

Next, I was given one of two choices: Prednisone or immunoglobulin (IVIg). We opted for the Prednisone which turned out to be terribly wrong. I have kidney stones which was aggravated, plus a development of diabetes. Prednisone is beneficial to some folks, though.

Well, this meant starting infusions of immunoglobulin. I am making some headway, but am aware as of now, we have no cure for IBM. However, we cannot give up on a cure one day in the future.

The best way I can describe my IBM symptoms are severe weakness, some pain, especially in my arms. Due to the multiple maladies, I get depressed, luckily, Zoloff is helping me to stay balanced.

I conclude with my personal way to cope with IBM. It is with the love from family and friends and prayers. Plus, we can always see someone else smiling through their own pain.

May God bless you to find your own way of copy with your Myositis disease.

IBM Case # 20

Male - Present Age 61

Dated Diagnosis:

(1) Wrong diagnosis in1975, Polymyositis

(2) Correct diagnosis in 1981 after a biopsy at Wellesky Hospital, Toronto, Ontario; the information from the founder, Dr. G. Karpeti, Montreal Neurologist Hospital Institute; the 'detective' work of my doctor J. Turley, Head of Neurology Laboratory, St. Michael's Hospital, Toronto, Ontario, and the work of the Head of Pathology, Dr. B. Bao at St. Michael's Hospital, Toronto, Ontario.

Medications:

16 mg Prednisone every other day for six months, then I have gradually reduced the amount to NOTHING, after taking it 25 years.

History:

I first noticed muscle weakness twenty-five years ago while I was working as an instructor at an athletic camp in Toronto, Ontario.

I was a Physical Educator teacher in the Toronto Public High School system and have always been a very active person.

Began having trouble running. I tired easily and my upper thigh muscles shrank.

The doctors in Toronto were mystified what I had and they thought it was Polymyositis and just put me on a heavy Prednisone schedule.

My condition stabilized for years but the disease came back with vengeance in 1991. My doctor, Dr. J. Turley, insisted I have another biopsy done at Wellesley Hospital

(NOTE: I had two previous biopsies, but improper staining of the muscle tissue had prevented a proper diagnosis)

Thanks to the good doctor (Turley) and the Pathologist at St. Michael's Hospital (Dr. Bao), the disease was diagnosed as IBM.

I traveled to Montreal with my X-rays to Dr. Karpeti

(Montreal Neurological Hospital) who confirmed the diagnosis.

Since the early 1980's, I have had three bad attacks of IBM followed by years of calmness.

My IBM is different than most because it has not affected my lower arms or hands in any way.

I have also had no pain except for some joint aching due to muscle weakness.

I have been retired from teaching for five years and the absence of everyday stress has certainly helped my situation.

1.) Accessories used

A walker and 'drop foot' leg braces.

2.) Physiotherapy:

The use of the TENS machine (**T**ranscutaneous **E**lectrical **N**erve **S**timulator) has helped me regain strength in my shoulder, arm, and neck muscles.

3.) Magnetic Pads:

Those have reduced the ache in my elbows.

4.) Water Exercise:

Excellent for Isotonic
muscle work (the water must
be at least 90 degrees F).

I had to stop my swim program for two reasons:

A) The prevalence of "Athlete's Foot" at the public pool.

B) The dressing room benches are too low for me to get up easily.

5.) Walking:

I now can walk over one mile per week using my walker.

6.) Isometric Exercise:

Every morning I do a set of resistance exercises for my upper arms and shoulder.

7.) Supplements:

Herb, (Pau d'Arco) which I have taken for 15 years and strongly feel it has reduced the inflammation.

500 mg Magnesium, Calcium and Zinc daily to enhance muscle contraction and string-thin-bone.

Creatine Monohydrate - 8 grams daily of this pure crystalline substance with water..

I started in October 1999 after Dr. Turley had sent me a

scientific article by Drs. Tarnopolsky & Bourgeois from the Hamilton, Ontario Medical Center.

I believe this study by these two Hamilton doctors is the first study of the therapeutic effect of Creatine on Myositis patients.

After one month of following the dosage that the Hamilton group of 91 patients used, I have had some dramatic and positive physiological changes.

I have muscle regene-ration and enlargement in my lower and upper legs, thighs and biceps; chest and shoulder muscles.

I have also had more energy and. therefore, want to exercise more frequently.

I now have been taking the replacement supplement for over six months weekly and still have less dramatic, but positive, muscle changes.

It has been amazing!!!

There have been no side effects and my doctor checks my progress every six months.

If you are interested, contact James R. Kilpatrick -JRKilpatrickMYO@aol.com.

He can send you the seven page study done by the Hamilton doctors.

- David W. Kent 4003 Bayview Ave, Apt. #311
North York, Ontario. Canada

IBM Case # 21

Diagnosed 1989
Male - Present Age 68

I am a sixty-eight year old male who has lived with IBM at least fourteen years. The first symptom was noticed in 1986 when unexpected weakness in my left arm almost caused me to drop a load I was carrying with both arms.

Subsequent examination and limited tests by a Rheumatologist failed to identify the cause of my difficulty.

Later, through a multiple series of electrical tests by a Neurologist and a biopsy of my right biceps, positive diagnosis was obtained in 1989.

It was again confirmed by an independent second opinion in 1990. In both cases, the doctors stated that no effective treatment for IBM was available.

In the early stages, as the disease progressed to both arms, the disabling effects were minimal, but the psychological impact was significant.

Until 1994, I knew of nobody with this rare and incurable disease and felt very much alone and depressed.

However, in 1994 two events happened which were instrumental in lifting my spirits and providing a basis for a more positive attitude.

First, I was fortunate to qualify for a trial at NIH (involving IVIg and Prednisone) where I met about ten other participants. Interchange of our experiences was both informative and comforting because I now realized that I was not alone, but had company for much needed support.

Second, I learned about the existence of an organization, the Myositis Associate of America (MAA), which is dedicated to helping people with IBM, PM and DM.

As a member, my sphere of acquaintances with IBM expanded tremendously, and the wealth of information about the disease and coping methods distributed by MAA were immeasurably beneficial.

As the disease continued to progress, coping with physical disability, using mechanical aids became necessary.

With increasingly weak legs, rising from a seated position or climbing stairs or walking any distance became very difficult, or even dangerous, without support.

* I now use firm cushions to elevate chairs

* A riser for the commode

* A cane for walking short distances

* A 4-wheeled rolling walker with hand brakes for longer distances

* A portable half-step for navigating steps.

* In 1997 I bought a van to eliminate the struggle required to get in and out of a standard car, and in anticipation of eventually needing a van to transport a scooter or power chair.

* With weak hands and fingers, Good-Grips utensils make eating a lot easier and thick-bodied pens/pencils help make my writing legible.

In addition, in lieu of any effective medical treatment, I have found that a regular program of appropriate physical exercises helps maintain flexibility and strength which translates to a more positive mental attitude as well.

But my best support comes from my wonderful wife who, for me, has given the word "caregiver" new meaning and appreciation.

For my benefit and hers, we are now planning to build a handicapped-accessible, single level house so we can better cope with any future challenges created by this insidious disease.

- Bill Babyak, Pennsylvania

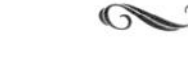

IBM Case # 22

Diagnosed 1988
Male -

At age 47 I noticed that I wasn't as strong as I used to be. After going to my doctor to get a physical, he had noted that my SGOT and LDH and Triglycerides were elevated and he did not know why.

After I had fallen several times, I went to my doctor and explained to him about my legs buckling. He examined me again and said my enzymes were abnormal and I may have Muscular Dystrophy. He sent me to a Neurologist and he diagnosed me as having Polymyositis and wanted to run more tests.

He sent me to have an EMG test. The doctor who

administered it concluded that I may have ALS.

I was then sent to have a muscle biopsy. The surgeon confirmed that I had an Inflammatory Myopathy (Poly-myositis). Then I was sent to the University of Virginia Medical School to see if I should be kept on Prednisone which I had been on awhile.

In February 1989, I was sent to Duke University for another examination to see if I should be put on another medication. They agreed with my first doctor that I should be kept on the same meds.

May 4, 1990, my first doctor went on a leave of absence and closed his office. This left me to seek help somewhere else. Not sure where to turn, we contacted the Multiple Sclerosis office. They put us in contact with the Muscular Dystrophy Association.

We got in touch with the Muscular Dystrophy office and registered with them and went to their clinic. Fortunately, I saw a doctor who knew a little bit about what I had and recommended a study that was going on at the National Institute of Health in Bethesda, Maryland. He got me on protocol for the program.

On my first appointment at NIH, they did a muscle biopsy and found that I had Inclusion Body Myositis. I had to be taken off the Prednisone as that was doing more harm than good. I started on the infusions of Immunoglobulin (IVIg) study.

The study was done in intervals for three months. There was no signs of me regaining any strength after the infusions were complete.

In 1992, I finally got off Prednisone. May 19-20, 1993 I went back to NIH for testing. I had a Barium swallow test that required me to swallow a radioactive solution that NIH studied. On the second day the doctors did an MRI scan from the forearms down. After this test was concluded, I went through an EMG test. This would conclude our time at NIH. I made the decision not to return to do any more testing due to the fact the last two tests were very uncomfortable.

March 24, 1997 I was measured for a new motorized wheel chair because I could no long maneuver the manual wheel chair.

On April 8, 1997 I began seeing a new Neurologist. He prescribed 300 mg/d of Neurontin caps (this is used for ALS patients with convulsions and was just released by the FDA). He ordered me to begin physical therapy for six sessions.

In April 1997 a home nurse from Olstein came to evaluate me for Physical Therapy. The nurse provided a shower physical therapist. and occupational therapy. This lasted six weeks.

May 27, 1997 I visited with the Neurologist and he increased my meds to 400 mg and would increase them each week until I had reached 1200 mg to see what happens.

May 30, 1997 I visited the Neurologist to have another EMG test. After this past visit we only went to see the Neurologist every six months. In September of 1997, I was put on Rilutek for six months. We could not tell if this drug had made any progress.

During the early months after being sent from doctor to doctor and no one had any straight answers. All we knew was that we were almost alone in this. The MDA gave us help with wheelchairs and no information on IBM. It was very discouraging, upsetting, and very frustrating. Having to go on disability at age 51 was devastating to me and my family - especially when they noticed my body slowly deteriorating.

We had to build a suitable house for my needs. Some things are better and some things are not. My wife and I are making the best of what we have now. She has become my caregiver and tends to all my many needs. This has become a real challenge for us.

It has been 12 years now. We try to have a positive outlook on our situation, because life is very short. However, it has taken us a very long time to get to this stage. We still have a long way to go!

- Warren A. Rumpf
108 Downing Drive
Chesapeake, Virginia 23322-8736
E-Mail: warrenrumpt@juno.com.

IBM Case # 23

Diagnosed April 1996
Male

Here is my story for the book. I hope you will find it useful.

I was diagnosed with Inclusion Body Myositis in April of 1996, although my symptoms began several years earlier.

I used to be a long distance runner. My first indication that something was wrong was a decline in the line running performance. This decline began in the mid 1980's. For instance, my running speeds declined from eight minute miles to 12 minute miles from 1985 to 1995. This was despite continuing to train by running an average of 30-40 miles a week.

I brought this problem to the attention of my doctor in 1990. He misdiagnosed it as Thyroiditis. By 1995 I could no longer rise from a crouching positions without using some form of support. Also, I became aware that I could not rise from a chair without pushing down on the arm rests.

Since I had already seen a doctor about my weakness, I simply ignore these symptoms. In January 1996, I mentioned them symptoms of a doctor in an urgent care center. Although I was there for something completely unrelated, the doctor was sharp enough to realize that I had a potentially serious muscle or neurological problem.

She did a preliminary neurological exam and then referred me to a Neurologist. The Neurologist did the usual series of tests including X-rays, electromyogram (EMG), a full spine MRI, and then sent me to the University of California at San Diego Medical Center.

There, the Neurologist gave me a preliminary diagnosis of IBM, which was confirmed with a muscle biopsy. That was in April, 1996.

At that time, I discussed treatment options with a Neurologist at UCST. I had read enough to know there were no proven treatments for IBM and the treatments usually prescribed and a variety of unpleasant or dangerous side effects.

I told the doctor I would prefer no treatment at all under those conditions. He agreed that this might be the best course of action.

So far, I am pleased that I made the decision to avoid drug therapies. Other than the muscle weakness, my health continues to be very good.

In 1988, two years after the diagnosis, I began falling quite frequently. Two of those falls resulted in fractures. One gave me a head injury.

At that time, I decided to be very aggressive with any equipment standpoint. Over the next year-and-a-half, I purchased a walker, full leg braces with crutches, a scooter and ultimately a power wheelchair.

Using these medical aids has eliminated the falls that I was suffering and, I believe, helped extend my mobility by avoiding over-stressing my knees and avoiding falls.

It has been my experience that injuries cause a far more rapid loss of strength than does the disease on its own.

Recently, I have noticed a substantial decrease in finger strength, especially the tips of my fingers. This has caused me to stop working because my occupation was writing and I no longer have the strength or stamina in the fingers to type for any length of time.

I am now attempting to use voice recognition software however, it is slow and cumbersome and not at all suited for the kinds of writing I used to do. This story was written using voice recognition software and it took me many times longer to finish than it would have back when I typed.

Overall, despite the disease, I would have to consider my life to be quite good. We have a van with a scooter lift and use it to travel. I also use my scooter around our local community for grocery shopping, sightseeing or just enjoying the fresh air.

Recently, I have taken up watercolor painting. This seems to be an activity I can perform well despite my restricted mobility.

- Mike Shirk

15969-21 Avenida Villaha San Diego, CA 92128
mikeshirk@earthlink.net

IBM Case # 24

Diagnosed 1999
Female - Present Age 69

I am a white female, age 69 years of age. I was diagnosed with IBM in 1999.

About the middle of the '90s, I began to notice a weakness in my thighs. I began having trouble getting up out of chairs. I had to use my arms to push myself up, then I began to fall, would just be walking and suddenly I was on the floor or the ground. I fell more inside the house.

I learned to compensate, like taking smaller steps, watch for drop of foot or uneven, low places, not to climb stairs without rails to hold on to, wearing walking shoes.

I searched several years for a doctor that could help me. I saw six or more doctors who had no idea what was causing the problems I had.

Finally, I talked my family doctor into doing a MRI on my spine to see if that was my problem. The doctor seemed to think I had a bad disc, so I saw a surgeon, had CAT scan dye test and the works, but my back was not the problem.

The surgeon sent me to see Dr. Aziz Shaibani at the Houston Neuro Clinic, 6624 Fannin Street, Suite 1670, Houston, TX 77230.

He did a biopsy in December, 1999 and found I had Inclusion Body Myositis (IBM). I began immune globin injections (IVIg) February 29, 2000.

I know it has helped me because I am now much stronger. I have not fallen in two months, get up from chairs with less problems, walk up stairs. I now can walk 3-4 miles five days a week and ride my bicycle.

I have no pain, do not walk with a walker or cane. I am so blessed

I am a nurse and I still work part time as a substitute at our schools and also sub for the nurses at an allergy clinic.

We made a 1,500 mile trip May 2, 2000 and I drove every mile.

Dr. Kilpatrick, you have my permission to use my name, address, etc. or delete any of this if you need to.

- Glenna Morlan

114 N. Mahan Drive

Richwood, TX 77531

(Editor's Note: Dr. Aziz Shaibani has been a tremendous supporter for the production of this book. He is also Director of the Nerve & Muscle Center of Texas, Houston. The Center was the first to place a larger order for the pre-published books.)

Thank you, Inclusion Body Myositis friends, for taking the time to express your thoughts and experiences so that other IBM diagnosed individuals may learn from you.

Chapter 4

JUVENILE DERMATOMYOSITIS

Juvenile idiopathic inflammatory myopathy (JIIM) or Juvenile Myositis (JM) most often presents itself as Dermatomyositis (JDM) with its typical rashes and muscle weakness. There are fewer cases of Juvenile Polymyositis (JPM), Inclusion Body Myositis (JIBM) and other clinical forms of Myositis reported.

The JDM rash precedes muscle weakness greater than 50% of the time. In both cases, (JPM and JDM) muscle weakness usually develops over a period of months, weeks, or days. The weakness being proximal (closest to and within the trunk of the body) primarily involves neck, hip, trunk and shoulder muscles, but may also include distal muscles Dysphagia (difficulty swallowing), Dysphonia (hoarseness), abdominal pain and arthritis can also occur with this disorder. Muscle pain is seen in approximately 50% of children with Myositis.

Corticosteroids are effective with complete withdrawal of medication can be anticipated in a large percentage of patients. Patients with severe weakness may need longer periods of treatment. For those patients who experience dose-limiting side effects of corticosteroids or are unresponsive, there are other treatments available, including intravenous immunoglobulin infusions (IVIg).

It is important to diagnose these patients and start treatment as soon as possible. The parents and the doctor of a child with Myositis will also want to consider a rehabilitation program with a team of professional experts in this field.

JDM - Case # 1

Diagnosed 3/6/98 at Age 7 Female - Present Age 9

JULIA'S STORY

By Ralph Becker, Julia's Father

Julia, like most kids in the winter in New England, caught a cold. As she recovered from it, she started to get a strange rash. First, her eyelids took on a pinkish-purplish color, then it spread to her joints - knuckles, elbows, knees, etc.

Julie was feeling some minor fatigue. Nothing you'd associate with any disease, at least not a disease anyone has heard of. Just a little more tired than normal.

Her pediatrician called it "Fifth Disease" and said it should go away within a few weeks. It didn't.

The next pediatrician who saw her got it right, and referred us to a Dermatologist, who sent us to Children's Hospital in Boston.

The doctors took blood, gave Julia an MRI, and performed a thorough clinical exam and declared it a positive diagnosis. Her rash was "classic" for the disease. They also detected a bit of weakness in her neck muscles.

Julia was put on 40 mg/d of oral Prednisone. Soon, thereafter, 200 mg/d of Plaquenil for the rash. Within a few weeks, most of her blood results returned to near normal. She was also starting to suffer the side effects of Prednisone - extreme moodiness, weight gain, "moon face," and so on. We began to slowly taper her off the Prednisone. As we did, her lab numbers began to creep up again.

Late that summer, Julia got a bit of a sunburn. We'd been using sun screen every day, but we were out of it one day, and she apparently didn't use enough of it.

The sunburn was not severe, but it's effects were.

It turns out that sun exposure can cause a flare (relapse) of JDMS. Julia's lab results spiked up, and we had to increase her Prednisone to compensate.

Her labs eventually returned to near normal again, but this time as we tapered Prednisone, her lab results increased in almost a direct correlation.

Over the next 8 or 9 months, we gradually decreased Julia's Prednisone and simultaneously added another oral drug to compensate: Methotrexate. At one point for several weeks, Julia was actually off of Prednisone. However, she was also growing more and more fatigued and started exhibiting signs of muscle weakness.

She had a series of falls and lacked the stamina to even spend the day at a zoo or an amusement park.

In June 1999, just after the school year ended, this decline culminated in a big spike in her lab results, the biggest thus far.

We hospitalized Julia for a 3-day course of steroid infusions, and some physical therapy. After being released, she took weekly infusions for most of the rest of the summer. She also began getting Methotrexate by injection every week.

This series of infusions and injections proved to be the key in getting Julia well again. As she improved, both in strength and stamina, we tapered the infusions from weekly to every two weeks, then every three weeks, eventually discontinuing them by the year of 1999.

Early in 2000, Julia had a school yard fall and broke her arm. This was probably partially due to a side effect of Prednisone for so long, depleting her body's calcium supply. Since then, she also takes calcium supplements to prevent this from happening again.

Since discontinuing her infusions, we have gradually tapered Julia's Prednisone, but this time her lab and clinical results have actually improved over time. Each new test shows her to be stronger and stronger.

By the spring of 2000, she's back to 100% muscle strength and endurance. We will take the next several months to continue tapering her medicine as long as the good results continue.

The doctors have even started using the "R-Word," Remission. We pray that they are right and the Diary can have a happy ending sooner, rather than later.

Julia's rash has been very tenacious throughout all the treatments. It is the most persistent rash our doctors have ever seen in a JDMS patient. The Plaquenil that she has been taking for nearly two years seemed to be having no effect.

We discontinued it and started a different drug, Quinacrine, that has shown very encouraging results in Europe. Finally, within the past few months, her rash has slowly started to get better. It's nearly to the point where it isn't even noticeable any more.

The whole journey is chronicled online in a Diary format. This Diary has brought us together in spirit with literally hundreds of other JDMS kids around the world. We've also met some wonderful people because of it. Through the Diary, Julia has become a great example for these families, and is arguably the most famous JDMS patient in the world.

Throughout the ordeal, Julia has shown an extraordinary level of courage. She has endured more pills and needles than most people will see in their lifetime.

Through it all, she has maintained excellence in school and her characteristic good spirits. She is not down on anyone about it and her faith has shown through like a beacon in the night.

We are incredibly proud of her,

Editor's Note: Everyone with a Myositis disease is happy that Julia has passed through a Myositis fire and has come out without being sieged. Thank you, Ralph Becker for submitting Julia's story.

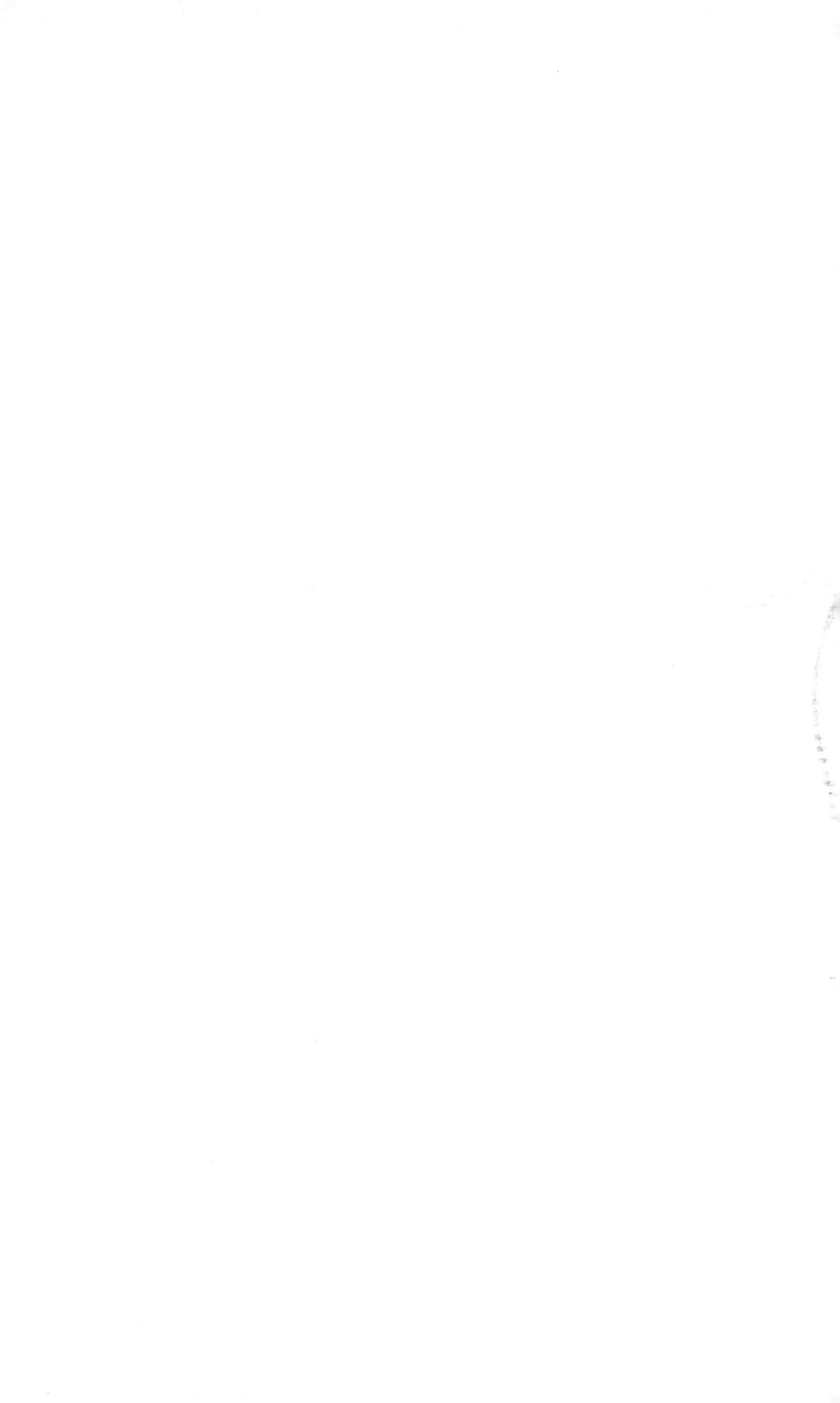